Overcoming Teacher Burnout in Early Childhood

Overcoming Teacher Burnout in Early Childhood

Strategies for Change

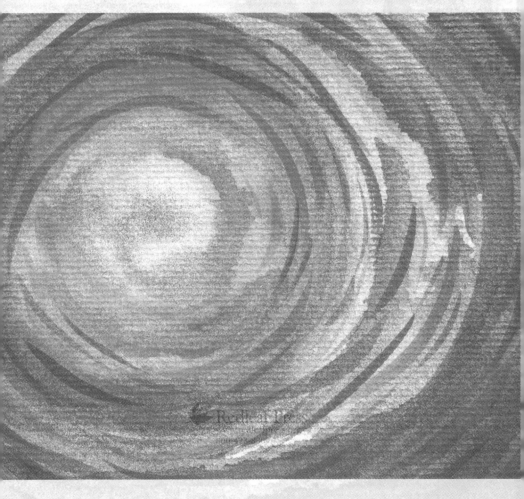

Ellen M. Drolette

Published by Redleaf Press
10 Yorkton Court
St. Paul, MN 55117
www.redleafpress.org

First edition 2019
Cover design by Jim Handrigan
Cover image by iStock.com/Benjavisa
Interior design by Jim Handrigan and Douglas Schmitz
Typeset in Mrs. Eaves
Printed in the United States of America
25 24 23 22 21 20 19 18   1 2 3 4 5 6 7 8

Library of Congress Cataloging-in-Publication Data
CIP data is on file with the Library of Congress.

Printed on acid-free paper

To my biggest cheerleaders and supporters, who are the inspiration for my passion in early education. Toddie, Dylana, Zach, Joanna, and sweet Nora Ellen, along with my amazing mom and dad: thank you.

Contents

Acknowledgments

Without the reliable flow of resources for early educators published by Redleaf Press, we would all be in a constant state of wondering what we need to do next. I would like to thank Redleaf Press and its excellent staff from the bottom of my heart: Laurie Herrmann, who got the ball rolling; Kara Lomen, who found me, planted a seed, watered it, let me work through the process with patience and understanding, and helped me make a dream come true; and Christine Zuchora-Walske, my editor.

Thank you to Roger and Bonnie Neugebauer not only for being incredible global role models but also for mentoring me as a new writer through *Exchange* magazine. Without that opportunity, this book would not exist.

Christine, Colleen, Traci, Libby, Elise, Laura, Renee, Angie, Stephanie, Heidi, Leighanne, Trisha, Betsy, Beth, Carly, Nicole, and Paula, I can't thank you enough for sharing your stories. All of you shared some difficult stories with me, and those stories opened some old wounds, causing some (hopefully cathartic) tears. These stories also provided opportunities to reflect on the goodness and light you bring to this world. Keep doing the excellent work with children and families that you do, and don't forget to take time for yourselves.

Ellen L. G., Emily S., Steve G., and Carly M., the Life Is Good Kids Foundation has given me a fantastic outlook on life. This was not my goal when I set out meeting and training with this bunch, but I gained more than I intended: lifelong friends, a new perspective on adverse childhood experiences, and best of all, optimism. When life gives me lemons, I "goodify" the heck out of them, add some sugar, fill that glass up with ice and water, and have a drink!

Thank you, Lisa G., for being my business partner and ongoing collaborator in Positive Spin, LLC. I am forever grateful for your continual creativity, enthusiasm, and confidence.

Last but certainly not least, I want to acknowledge my family, who have been my biggest cheerleaders since the beginning. To my husband, Todd: thank you for putting up with my glares and sarcasm when I was typing away and did not hear you asking me questions. Thank you for always being my sounding board and taking all my grandiose ideas and varied emotions without judgment. To my kids, Dylana and Zach: you inspire me every day. Never underestimate the value of relationships in the work you do. They matter. To Mom and Dad: thanks for being my editors since I learned to write, for listening to me read different sections of this book, and for always lifting my confidence when I needed it most. Most of all, thank you for always knowing that I *could* when I thought I could not. You are indeed the best parents ever. To my sister and brother, Leigh and Joseph, you're not bad either—I will keep you. I love you all.

Introduction

I AM AN EARLY CHILDHOOD EDUCATOR. Some people balk at calling family child care providers *early childhood educators*. For many of my years as a family child care provider, the lack of respect for my position made me feel like a bottom-feeder in the early education world. I felt that I ranked lower than my peers who worked in special education, center-based programs, or public schools. It took me many years to realize that all of us doing this job are fighting the same fight. We are all trying to get children and families what they need to be successful. Negativity about the work I do; about my own self-worth; and about the lack of advocacy for children, families, and early education as a whole is a burden that not only I but many early educators have carried. This burden contributes to stress, burnout, and low morale for all kinds of early educators—not just family child care providers.

My Story

I have been exploring stress, burnout, and low morale in the field of early education for twenty-five years. The beginning of my story as an educator is important because this profession was not my life plan. A career in early childhood education had never entered my mind.

1

My professional life started out in dentistry. I had an excellent full-time job as a dental assistant and front office coordinator. I enjoyed it immensely. I was fulfilled, I felt appreciated, I found the work challenging and interesting, and I had built strong friendships. What more could I want from my profession?

During my time as a dental assistant, from the mid-1980s to the early 1990s, I became plagued by constant sneezing, upper respiratory issues, and skin woes. At that time, all the dentists, hygienists, and assistants used powdered latex gloves. When the staff would remove their gloves, the powder would explode into the air, which would cause me to break out in hives and become a sneezy, blotchy-faced mess. My allergist confirmed what we all feared: I was severely allergic to latex, and my allergy was not going to get better. In fact, repeatedly exposing an allergic person to this type of allergen just worsens the symptoms.

In an attempt to reduce my symptoms, I began working only at the front desk. My days started out well. I would come in mostly clearheaded each morning. (But I was never entirely clearheaded because allergies are cumulative; every exposure makes the allergy a little worse.) Usually by midday my eyes would become bright red, and I would start sneezing. The more movement there was in the office and the more dentists and hygienists were working, the worse I would react. I would arrive home each night after work exhausted, with hands so irritated that only immersing them in ice water would relieve them.

In the meantime, I had gotten married, had my first child, and placed her in child care. I had to go back to work six weeks after giving birth. I had no paid maternity or family leave. Someone else in the office had to work sixty to seventy hours a week to cover my maternity leave. When I did return, I had no place to pump breast milk, and my time was ruled by the dentists' schedules.

When our daughter was a year old, my husband and I found out we were expecting our son. While I was home on maternity leave with him, I had eight weeks of healthy breathing and skin. This respite helped me realize that my allergies had become a hindrance to my everyday life. At work I could not get through a conversation without sneezing three times. I came home from work completely wiped out. In addition, my child care was mediocre at best, and I was making just enough to pay for child care and groceries. My husband and I reevaluated our finances and our life balance. We decided that it was time to change the course of our family life. We determined that I would return to work at the dental office in January 1994 to give an eight-week notice. I would start a family child care program in mid-March 1994.

I left the job I loved with a heavy heart and many tears. However, I was ready to take back my health and set out on a new adventure. I had big plans for my child care program. I was going to be way better than "mediocre at best." I was not going to be any of the things that I hated as a working parent with her child in child care. I was going to be an excellent communicator. I would never close without sufficient notice. I would follow all the rules. These things I knew. I was very sure of myself.

Here are some real-life facts I found out quickly about my new career that first year:

PERCEPTION: I thought I was going to do child care temporarily to meet the financial needs of my family, and when both children went off to kindergarten, I would get a different job.

REALITY: Well, that didn't happen. I did meet my family's financial needs, but I also discovered that child care was more than a job. This work was a profession. I learned that I could advocate for children and families, feel empowered, and be a real leader. Like many early childhood educators, I didn't see myself as an advocate right away. It took time. But once I found my voice, I didn't want to give it up.

PERCEPTION: I thought I would not fall in love with other people's children.

REALITY: Boy, was I wrong! I have fallen in love with every child who has walked through my door. It is impossible for me not to fall in love with the children in my care when I spend forty-plus hours each week with them, watching them grow and learn. So there. I am going to love the children. I am going to get attached to them, and hopefully they will connect with me. Children need to have healthy attachments with adult caregivers.

PERCEPTION: I vowed that I would be better than mediocre, because I know what a working parent goes through emotionally and physically.

REALITY: I think I succeeded. I was (and am) better than mediocre. I think we can all strive for that by starting small and simply aiming above the average.

PERCEPTION: I thought that taking care of my own kids would be a piece of cake.

REALITY: It wasn't. In fact, my own children were probably the most stressful to care for. They owned me, and they were not going to let anyone else hold their real estate. They were kind to other children. They shared their belongings and had their space to escape. It's just that I was stretched thin, and they knew that. It was hard on them, and it was hard on me. I was new in my field and had no experience. When my kids went to elementary school, my job got easier.

PERCEPTION: I thought that anyone could do child care.

REALITY: They can't. They really, really cannot! No! It takes a special combination of personality, skills, and knowledge. It would have helped me a lot if I had taken child development courses before opening my program. That would have given me a better understanding of all the needs my children were experiencing.

It is no wonder I have learned what burnout is. I guess that's what I get for going into early education with no experience, thinking I had it all figured out.

I know better now. I eventually realized it was imperative for me to get my Child Development Associate (CDA) credential, so that families would feel reassured that I knew a little something about child development. This credential proved that I had some knowledge. I became more and more involved in local associations, networks, and state-level meetings, which helped tremendously in building my knowledge. Over time I became well educated and began to really understand why kids do the things they do. I learned early childhood theory and practice and the importance of being a lifelong learner.

About twenty-five years later, I am still here. My children went off to kindergarten, high school, college, careers, and marriage. I went back to school later in life to get my bachelor's degree in human services with a focus on early childhood education from Springfield College.

Throughout my early childhood education career, I have felt burnout and low morale many times. I am a small business owner, and I am the sole proprietor. I have a responsibility to support my family through good times and bad. My husband and I are both self-employed. My husband owns a construction company. At the height of the Great Recession back in 2008, life was difficult for us, but my salary proved to be imperative. I was unhappy during that period in my life. I was tired. I never looked forward to my days with children.

What is more, living and working through the seasons in Vermont is no easy feat! Vermont has five distinct seasons: autumn, winter, mud season, spring, and summer. Winter is the longest season. The days are short, and the weather is cold through late April. Although Vermont has glorious landscapes, it is not for the fainthearted or thin-blooded. The prolonged lack of sunlight and the cold are hard to handle sometimes.

When I am getting burned out, everything is a chore (including caring for the children I love), and nothing seems right (including the weather). If I start to feel this way, I know that something needs to change.

About seven years ago, I finally found the right formula to keep my fire lit. It consists of wellness, education, balance, and optimism. I didn't figure this out quickly or easily. It has been a journey that has fulfilled me in unexpected ways. I have met remarkable, empowering people who have changed how I view myself and how I live each day. I have learned that I have choices in my life. I have chosen to stay close to those who inspire me, make me laugh, see my potential, and push me to be a better version of myself. I have also seen a therapist, and that relationship has helped me understand how important perception is. How others perceive a situation and how I perceive it might not agree, and neither is necessarily true. This slight shift in my thinking has been essential to my growth. I've learned that boosting my own morale and avoiding burnout requires a multifaceted approach.

The Problem of Teacher Burnout

In the teaching profession, and many other professions that deal directly with people, we often hear, "I am just so burned out from this job." I have heard this more times than I can count. I have even uttered these words myself. But what is burnout?

I turned to *Psychology Today* for a definition. "Burnout is not a simple result of long hours. The cynicism, depression, and lethargy of burnout can occur when you're not in control of how you carry out your job, when you're working toward goals that don't resonate with you, and when you lack social support. If you don't tailor your responsibilities to match your true calling, or at least take a break occasionally, you could face a mountain of mental and physical health problems" (Sussex Publishers, accessed 2018).

Early in my career, I noticed that caregiver fatigue and stress were high and morale was low in many settings. No matter the type of program—large or small, center or family child care, private or public, parochial or nonprofit, nanny or franchise—the work is tough physically and mentally.

The pay grade for early educators tends to be low, increasing the stress in their personal lives, and this stress can overflow into the classroom. In addition to low pay, the physical and mental demands of the job combined with lack of self-care and lack of professional and emotional support are significant causes of burnout.

The feeling of being cared for, appreciated, and respected can lift morale in a matter of seconds. However, early childhood educators often feel ignored, underappreciated, and disrespected. They have trouble mustering the energy it takes to continue in the field. Some leave early childhood education. Others keep going anyway because early childhood educators have a passion for bettering the lives of young children. But when they stay on in a burned-out state of mind, they are not fostering high-quality outcomes for children. Adults are responsible for delivering high-quality experiences to children; the stakes are high. So what is a burned-out educator to do?

In my role as a CDA professional development specialist, I conduct interviews with candidates. One question on an old version of the interview was "Knowing that fatigue can be high and morale can be low in this field, what do you do to care for yourself?" I usually chose this question to ask because the answers were so revealing. This question was often met with a blank stare, silence, and then grasping for words. Candidates would say, "Well, I take long showers when I can," or "I try to get seven hours of sleep every night." I became accustomed to answers based on necessities of daily living rather than higher-level self-care (Drolette 2016).

Self-care is just the tip of the iceberg. Supervision, peer networking, professional therapy, and support groups are necessary for combating burnout. With guidance and reflection, early childhood educators can make reasonable changes in their personal and professional lives to get past the bumps in the road. Preventing and overcoming burnout is crucial not only for our own well-being but also for the well-being of the children and families in our programs.

How This Book Can Help You

In this book, I share lots of personal stories and conversations. I want the book to reflect reality as closely as possible. My relationships with the people in these stories and conversations lie at the heart of everything I've shared. I hope this relationship-based exploration makes the topic feel personally relevant and helps you understand how much relationships matter in this field and in life. The stories and conversations are real experiences of real people. I hope you find connection and comfort in that knowledge.

The stories come from a variety of child care providers who work in different settings. They have all had experiences that have led to negativity, depression, and burnout. These stories show how the educators persisted through low morale and moved from pessimism to optimism.

Optimism, gratitude, joy, and connection start from within and grow outward. They begin with a choice to improve your personal situation by making changes, either big or small. After each story, you will find a set of reflection statements or questions. Take some time to read and ponder these ideas.

Think critically about your own story as you read through this book. How you react to a complicated, stressful situation has everything to do with your own experiences. Do certain triggers make you think of episodes from your past? The knowledge you've gained from past experiences—good or bad—is the foundation upon which you make all your decisions.

This book is designed for use by peer groups of early childhood educators or leaders seeking both self-reflection and rich group conversation. As you read, highlight text that seems important. As you reflect, take notes on your thoughts and emotional reactions. If you like, talk about all these ideas with your peers or someone close to you.

Each story and suggestion will resonate differently with different educators. Each person has a way of dealing with stress and combating burnout. Some educators may need to use many coping techniques, and others may need only reminders. Feel free to share on my Facebook author page (Ellen M. Drolette) what has worked for you.

Once you've finished reading, pondering, and discussing this book, you have an important job to do. Ask yourself, "Am I carrying a lot of emotional baggage?" If the answer is yes, evaluate that baggage, drop what you can, and move on. You will continue to carry a certain amount of baggage; nobody can forget everything. But you should keep reevaluating throughout your lifetime. Through regular reflection, you can rid yourself of unnecessary burdens and keep growing and thriving as an early childhood educator.

CHAPTER 1

Work-Life Balance

Christine's Story: Struggling to Find Work-Life Balance

Christine worked at a large nonprofit child care program in an administrative role. When I first met her, her morale was low and she felt stuck in her job. She had been offered another position elsewhere at a lower wage but with much less stress. Christine loved her job and adored her students. She felt torn between staying or leaving.

Christine supervised two teachers. These teachers wanted her to fix things that she couldn't fix. The program had rules restricting teachers during breaks and lunch. The organization did not have enough qualified teachers to fill all positions, so it constantly shuffled staff to comply across all its program locations. Because of these ongoing coverage issues, teachers could not leave the center during breaks or lunch. Christine's staff often complained to her. But she had no control over the staffing regulations or the center's rules. This problem was not only bringing down teacher morale, but it was also increasing stress on supervisors, who had to cope with the low morale but couldn't do anything about its cause. Christine tried to boost staff morale by bringing the teachers their favorite muffins or doing yoga classes with them. Christine offered a shoulder for them to cry on. She listened, gave advice, and provided support.

But Christine herself felt unsupported. She admitted that she felt dumped on. Getting out of bed and going to work had become a chore. After working nine hours each day, she was taking classes four nights a week. She was feeling fried. Her fire was burning out.

Christine had an ongoing desire to make sure that children were getting 100 percent of the attention and support they needed from the teachers and that the teachers were getting what they needed from her. But, she wondered, what good are the staff to children if the adults are tired and overworked?

This situation was detrimental to Christine's well-being. She explained, "I don't have any balance of work and life. I barely have time to breathe. I also have a disabled brother who lives with us and needs a lot of care." Christine said her saving grace was going to church weekly. Christine felt that attending church gave her time to clear her mind and start her week with a fresh perspective. She also tried to practice yoga. She knew she benefited from yoga, but she sometimes had difficulty getting there. She was exhausted. She faced a conundrum. She knew that going to yoga would help her, but she had so much to get done.

It's Hard to Share from an Empty Cup

Stories like Christine's are familiar to most early childhood educators. They are playing out all over the country. They are tales of low pay, family needs, flagging mental health, lack of self-care, low morale and confidence, frustration, and, in family child care, isolation. Educators have good days and bad days, but when work and life are out of balance, the bad days seem to take over.

We want to spend time with our own families, but we also need to meet our professional development requirements, run a business, take care of ourselves, and try not to miss work because finding a substitute is really, really hard. It is a harsh reality that everything outside of the actual care and teaching of children has to be done in the evening. How do we make meals for our family, exercise regularly, assess, plan, conference, clean, organize, learn, care, hug, love, and clean some more when there are only twenty-four hours in a day? It is a lot. We end up having to make difficult choices. Is it even possible to find a healthy balance as professionals in the field of early childhood care and education?

As an early childhood educator myself, I can relate to Christine's struggles. I like to use the metaphor "my cup is full" when my sense of well-being has been boosted by having a good day with children, attending a decent training, listening to live music, or being the lucky recipient of a sweet gesture from someone else. That metaphorical cup can start leaking if my personal needs go unmet. For example, taking four nights of training in a week—or skipping my yoga class or my morning walk—drains my cup little by little. Before long, my cup is empty. There's nothing left to give. That is when it becomes difficult to be a good spouse, parent, and friend. Something must change, because if this scenario continues, my personal and professional relationships will suffer.

I have realized that sometimes my sanity and well-being need to take priority—even if it means a financial setback. I have also come to realize how important it is to be present in each moment. A children's book titled *The Three Questions* by Jon J. Muth helped me understand the latter. It tells the story of a boy who wants to know how to always be a good person. He thinks that he'll be able to do this if he can find the answers to three questions: What is the best time to do things? Who is the most important one? and What is the right thing to do? The story illustrates in a poignant way that now is the most important time, because it is the only time when we have any power. The most important person is the one we are with, for we don't know if we will ever have dealings with anyone else. And the right thing to do is to do that person good.

Reflection

- What does your week look like when your work life and personal life are in balance and everything is going well?

- Are you using your time efficiently to meet your own needs as well as those of the people around you?

- How do you deal with the reality that some decisions are out of your control?

- If you are a supervisor, how do you handle the struggles teachers face in the classroom while coping with your own stressors? How can both roles be supported in your setting?

CHAPTER 2

Setting Priorities

Colleen's Story: Prioritizing What's Important

Colleen had been in the field of education for twelve years, in a variety of settings. She started her career as a teacher's aide in a public school. Later she became a licensed middle school teacher. Colleen would go home each day from the latter job and cry over the enormous amount of papers that needed correcting, curriculum that needed creating, and documentation that needed recording to keep up with the pace her employer expected.

The pressure eventually became overwhelming. Colleen realized she didn't share her employer's priorities. After six years in the public school system, she left. She had her first child and entered the field of early education.

She started her new career path at a preschool. This preschool had a strong focus on foreign language development and math skills. Students learned addition and subtraction of double digits and other academic lessons that most kindergartners barely touch. The director and owner would hover when Colleen was teaching. Their hovering made her feel that they did not trust her teaching abilities.

Once again, Colleen realized that her priorities were different from those of her employer. She left the preschool.

Colleen decided to start her own family child care and preschool program. She had finally found her niche as an educator, but she still struggled with prioritizing what was important to her. Documentation was one of the tasks that brought her down. The amount of documentation she had to do as a business owner was similar to the paperwork she'd done as a public school teacher. She found the time required for this task to be burdensome. She wondered if the benefits of documentation were worth the stress and whether there was some way to lighten the burden.

When I started talking to Colleen and asked her about burnout, her thoughts went straight to preventing burnout for families in her care by relieving stress for working families and those in crisis. She had done a lot of work with the Strengthening Families Framework. Strengthening Families is an approach to working with families that's meant to increase family strengths, enhance child development, and reduce the likelihood of child abuse and neglect. It is based on building parental resilience, social connections, and knowledge about child development and parenting; offering concrete family support; and building children's social and emotional competence. Colleen said she'd noticed that she, like many early childhood educators, often thought she was helping families when in fact she might have been enabling them by giving them help all the time instead of encouraging them to figure out ways to solve problems themselves—and burning herself out in the process. Colleen admitted that in the early days of running her program, she gave too much. She realized this was contributing to her stress level, and she had to pull back to have energy for her own two boys. Colleen's husband, a firefighter, was often gone on twenty-four-hour shifts. While they supported each other's professions, there wasn't enough give-and-take between professional and personal needs. Colleen saw that she could not continue to offer movie nights and date nights for families at the expense of her sanity.

Colleen told me about a day that was etched in her memory because it was one of those "worst days." A child who disliked napping kept climbing out of the crib. She had no opportunity to deal with any dishes or messes or take a breather. At the end of the day, she was standing at the sink starting to wash dishes when her husband walked in. He said, "Wow, what a mess. I don't know how you can stand this." She burst into tears because she was at her wits' end. Her husband realized the kind of day she was having about ten seconds too late. He backpedaled quickly.

Colleen was a vocalist. She used to participate in a vocal group every Tuesday night. It was her night to go out and sing, and she never missed it. She called it her "me night." Eventually the group members decided that they needed to practice two nights a week. As a business owner, young mom, and spouse, Colleen found it impossible to commit to that. She had a hard time letting go of this activity. It was an important piece of her self-care.

Colleen noticed that when she started to feel stressed and burned out, she spent more time on her phone. Her phone let her disconnect and escape easily. She fell into a negative pattern of not being fully present.

After describing her personal challenges, Colleen expressed grave concern for her profession as a whole: "The early childhood field, in general, is not in a good space. The field feels 'battered down.'"

CAREGIVERS TEND TO BE PEOPLE PLEASERS. Many people who are caregivers—including early childhood educators—find themselves defined by their role. It ends up consuming their entire lives, from the moment they wake up in the morning until they go to bed at night, sometimes six or seven days a week. When you are a caregiver, a people person, and a giver, it is easy to forget that your work is not the only thing in your world and that you need to do other things too, to feed your soul.

In James Patterson's novel *Suzanne's Diary for Nicholas*, a character says, "Imagine life is a game in which you are juggling five balls. The balls are called work, family, health, friends, and integrity. And you're keeping all of them in the air. But one day you finally come to understand that work is a rubber ball. If you drop it, it will bounce back. The other four balls . . . are made of glass. If you drop one of these, it will be irrevocably scuffed, nicked, perhaps even shattered" (Patterson 2001, 20–21).

Hobbies that make you happy and activities that are important to you are essential to your well-being. Hobbies, sports, church, clubs, and so on can be crucial self-care tools. You might not realize the importance of such activities until you aren't doing them anymore. You may start building up angst, and for some that leads to an internal combustion that manifests in a variety of harmful habits.

For example, when Colleen could not do her vocal group any longer, she filled that time with work or family obligations instead of self-care activities. When I became injured and could not participate in my running group, instead of finding another self-care activity to fill that time, I worked. Colleen and I—and all early childhood educators—need to be more mindful of how we are intentionally caring for ourselves. We need to set aside one or two nights per week or per month that are just for us.

When we're burned out, it becomes almost impossible to model patience. Sometimes it is hard even to smile. It's definitely hard to feel happy or to feel that we're doing a good job at anything.

This is a common problem for educators. While families are the focus of our work, work cannot be the sole focus of our lives. It is essential for us as educators to continually assess our priorities and our level of burnout. While you are holding space for others, find a way to hold space for yourself too. That might mean tweaking your morning and evening routines so they include time to stretch and breathe. It could also mean evaluating how you spend your work time so you are prioritizing the work you feel is most important and minimizing the work that drags you down.

Colleen has been figuring out the best ways for her to keep her priorities in order. When I asked her how she keeps grounded, she talked about a philosophy of simplicity and "white space." She said this philosophy helps her focus on what is essential in her life. She sent me an article that illustrated what the term *white space* means regarding the human psyche.

In this article, an interview with productivity expert Juliet Funt, Funt refers to white space as "the thinking time, the strategic pause that's in between the busyness" (Miller 2017). As I dove deeper into Funt's work around the idea of white space, I found myself inspired by the simplicity of this idea while simultaneously kicking myself for always working harder, not smarter. Funt says people no longer "value the idea of retreating into thought to find an idea that will turbo charge a business, or a company, or a project. That work is hard, and it's very advanced, and it requires quietness, and we're afraid of the quiet. Instead, we go to a new fuel source, the source of exertion, and we work hard, and we drive harder, and we log more hours, and we stay connected, and we feel as if exertion will replace the gems of thoughtfulness" (Miller 2017).

The idea of white space helped Colleen reflect on her priorities and streamline her paperwork duties. She established e-pay for tuition payments. This change has simplified her work life by eliminating the need to run to the bank.

Colleen mused, "There is only so much time in my life." She said that she has had to identify what she likes and wants to do as choices, and that she must consciously choose not to say yes to everything. She found herself running down the list of what needed to get done in the leadership team she facilitates, and she noticed that her name was next to all the tasks. She realized that she needed to give up some tasks she has held on to for years, and she resolved to speak up about it. She realized that when meetings that were supposed to be helpful started feeling like they were hurting, it was time to reevaluate them.

Colleen read a plethora of professional articles and is always referring to them when speaking with her peers. She had a talent for remembering what she read and referring back to it. Through her reading, Colleen has gained invaluable tools for working with families as well as an understanding of what she needs, what the children in her care need, and how she can prioritize what's important

Many people use yoga class to ground themselves and to reconnect the body, mind, and spirit. Yoga therapy is different from a yoga class. Yoga therapy is typically used to seek out relief for a health condition. It is approached one-on-one with a specialist called a yoga therapist. Many people seek out yoga therapy for help sleeping and coping with stress, and as a general therapy alternative.

to create a better balance for her and her family. Colleen has also seen a yoga therapist, who has helped Colleen clear her mind and heart during stressful times.

●　●

Reflection

Juliet Funt recommends asking yourself the following four questions (Miller 2017):

- "Is there anything I can let go of?"
- "Where is good enough, good enough?"
- "What do I truly need to know?"
- "What deserves my attention?"

And I'll add one more question: "Is there time to be quiet in your day?"

CHAPTER 3

Coping with Setbacks

Traci's Story: A Tremendous Loss

Traci ran her own family child care program. She experienced a tremendous loss when the father of one of the children she had cared for since infancy passed away after a drawn-out battle with cancer. This family, like all the families she cared for, meant a lot to Traci. While Dad battled the disease, he still found the energy to visit Traci's program. Dad passed away after a long period of suffering.

After the father's death, Traci became the family's rock. She supported the mother and child far beyond what anyone would ever expect from a child care provider. This family was part of Traci's community. She was willing to do whatever she could to ease their pain.

One day when the child wasn't scheduled to come to Traci's house, Mom needed care for the child. Traci was already fully enrolled that day, but her seventeen-year-old daughter was home. So Traci had her daughter babysit the little one, and this kept her program in regulatory compliance. That day a state licensing inspector showed up. Traci explained why an extra child was there. She pointed out that her daughter was babysitting the child. While the inspector was present, another child had to go to the bathroom. Traci's daughter did what any helpful person would do and said, "I'll take him to the bathroom." And off she went with the child. At this moment, the inspector realized that Traci's program was out of compliance because the child was being cared for briefly by Traci's daughter, not Traci. Traci's families received a parent notification letter by mail a few days later. The letter stated that a serious violation had occurred. The state also posted the violation on Traci's program's online profile, where potential new families could see it. In addition, Traci had to post the letter in her program space for a specified period of time and have her families sign it.

Traci was devastated. She considered herself a rule follower. Furthermore, she was trying to help a family in great need, and she believed she had her bases covered. This small incident caused significant upheaval for Traci, both personally and professionally. She felt angry, sad, and deflated. She choked up with tears as she expressed her disappointment with the inspector's lack of understanding: "A child's father died!" She felt that the inspector could have chosen not to give a notice of serious violation. Given the chance, Traci could have corrected the situation immediately.

The inspector told Traci she could have gotten a variance to the enrollment rule. However, Traci's situation was unexpected, and variances take several weeks to receive. "Some things are not cut-and-dried when it comes to caring for people," she said. An appeals process was in place for issues like this, but Traci felt that an appeal would not have been worthwhile because there was a disconnect between the regulations and the reality of serving families. She explained, "I did not appeal because I felt like they just would not get it." She went on, "I would do it again. It was the right thing to do. Sometimes the right choice does not fit with the rule. It is not like we are stocking shelves. These are people's lives."

Traci felt emotionally zapped. She lost confidence and excitement in her work. She felt low and empty. She needed to feel empowered again, but she was unsure where to begin in building herself back up.

Loss, Mistakes, and Other Setbacks in Early Childhood Education

When I look back on losses I suffered and some decisions I made in the early part of my career—decisions I made for the good of the families—I wonder whether I made some mistakes. For example, one Friday in November 1999 I took the day off. My father was having surgery to remove an abdominal aneurysm. The hospital was a few hours away from home, and I thought it would be good to hang out with my mom and keep her occupied. My dad was coming out of his general anesthesia when I got a phone call.

The call was from my husband, back at home. He said that his mother was in the emergency room. She'd suffered an arrhythmia while she was attending a board meeting. The medical staff had gotten her heart rate back to normal in the ER and had her on life support, but things were not looking good. My dad was stable and in good hands, so I rushed back home.

My mother-in-law passed away that weekend. I was grieving. My husband was grieving. My young children were grieving too. However, I opened my family child care as usual on Monday because I did not want to inconvenience anyone. At the time, it seemed like the right thing to do. After all, I was going to have to close at the end of the week for services.

That week was probably one of the worst ones I've ever had. I cried a lot. The kids saw me cry, and their parents saw me cry. I should not have opened my program. I needed more time to grieve before I could begin healing and come back to work.

As early childhood educators, we know that when we take time off, it is a huge inconvenience—to us, to the children, and to the families. Finding a substitute can be next to impossible, especially for family child care programs. But we need to remember that we are human.

Grieving, Healing, and Starting Over

I was Traci's mentor and had been for quite some time. I wanted to take away all her heartache and hurt, as a mother would for her child. However,

I knew I had to let her experience the pain she felt, help her reflect on the journey that had brought her there, and help her learn from it.

First I tried to support Traci while she was unpacking all her emotion and frustration. After getting the notice of serious violation, Traci felt upset and hurt. She was adamant that she should stop participating in her state's Quality Rating and Improvement System (QRIS). (QRIS is a system of assessing, improving, and communicating the level of quality in early childhood and school-age care and education programs. QRIS awards quality ratings to programs that meet a defined set of standards.) Traci knew she was going to lose points in one of the QRIS areas, lowering her rating. She was disappointed in herself, and she decided that rather than face her mistake within the QRIS system, she would just not participate at all. I knew she had far more potential than she was giving herself credit for, but Traci needed time.

I interviewed Traci. As she told me the story of the family's tragedy and her licensing visit, I realized that Traci had not had the proper time to grieve for the dad who'd died. This man had not only been a parent in her program but had also grown up alongside her in the same neighborhood. I heard some anger in her voice. I let her unload her bitterness and rage. As I listened, I saw that Traci had been traumatized not only by the family's tragedy but also by how the state licensing agency handled her situation.

She exclaimed, "Was anyone worried about how I was doing? How the children were doing? How the family was doing? No one asked. I was a mess."

After Traci had processed her emotions, together we worked on her healing. I encouraged her to learn from her mistakes as well as others' mistakes. I explained that mistakes can make people feel angry, resentful, and bitter. I told her it's okay to feel those emotions, but afterward it's time to let them go—for everyone's sake. Cherishing negative emotions helps no one. I urged Traci to try to see the intention behind the licensing inspector's decision and turn the whole incident into a learning experience. This healing and learning took time and lots of self-talk.

Eventually Traci was able to pick up her self-confidence again and start rebuilding her program. She started attending professional network meetings on a regular basis. She built relationships with other family child care program owners. Eventually Traci became a leader, and she often shared her story with her peers. She learned, and she helped others learn, that asking for help is sometimes necessary when you are in a tough spot. And she realized that everyone makes mistakes. As George Bernard Shaw pointed out in the preface to his play *The Doctor's Dilemma*, "A life spent in making mistakes is not only more honorable but more useful than a life spent doing nothing" (Shaw 1911, lxxxv).

● ●

Reflection

- What angered Traci about the situation that occurred?
- What kind of support did the family in crisis get?
- What kind of support did Traci get?
- Do you think the licensing decision was helpful or harmful to Traci and the families in her care?
- How could Traci boost her confidence and let the world know that she indeed has what it takes to provide a high-quality program?
- What would you say to Traci if she were your peer?

CHAPTER 4

Compassion Fatigue

Libby's Story: Empathy Overload

Libby had a master's degree in early childhood education. When I met her, she had worked in the field for twelve years. She started out her career in a university-affiliated preschool and kindergarten program serving an affluent population. She remained at the program for six years. This program fostered Libby's understanding of typically developing children and diverse types of curriculum. Libby encountered no children who had experienced trauma. She never suffered low morale, received a lot of support, and enjoyed a highly professional atmosphere. The leadership was consistent, the pay was good, she received the same benefits and vacation time as the other university employees did, and the families valued her work.

Libby and her family moved several states away. She found a new job at a center as a floater covering lunches, breaks, teachers' prep times, and whatever other needs arose. Her first year was rough. The job came without benefits, and the director said she wasn't sure how long Libby would be in that position before one with benefits would open. She was a floater for a few months.

Then Libby became a long-term substitute for an assistant teacher who went on maternity leave. The head teacher in this classroom was young, had little experience, and lacked the necessary skills to lead the classroom. Several children who had experienced trauma were students in this classroom and weren't receiving the support they needed. Libby was not yet familiar with the resources in her new community, and she lacked authority in this classroom, so she couldn't offer much support herself. She grew more and more distressed with the head teacher's incompetence. The director took a medical leave, making the staffing situation dire. While Libby waited for the director's return, she observed and documented day-to-day happenings in the classroom and did what she could to support the children. When the director returned, she reviewed Libby's documentation and collected more information about the children's newly discovered needs. The director decided the head teacher did not have the skills required to run the classroom or to recognize the children's needs. She terminated that teacher, promoted Libby to head teacher, and hired a new assistant.

While Libby was trying to do the right thing, she never wanted or intended to get anyone fired. But that's what happened, and it created a painful, stressful situation for Libby. The parents of the children in the classroom were upset, and so were the other teachers in the center.

What is more, Libby found herself overwhelmed by the challenges of teaching at this center. Because of her experience at her first teaching job, Libby had lofty standards for herself as a teacher and for the program that now employed her. At her new job, she began to see that the population of families and the circumstances of the program could profoundly affect everyone's experience. At Libby's new job, many children had experienced trauma and had special physical, cognitive, and mental health needs. Several of her students were recent immigrants who had just started learning the English language. These English-language learners had parents with similar language barriers, making family communications difficult.

Libby had to reevaluate her classroom practice. She needed access to an early childhood Multi-Tier System of Supports (MTSS) for herself, her coteacher, and the children and families in her program. MTSS is a systematic way of identifying and supporting the needs of vulnerable children.

Libby described the low morale of the staff when she began working in the program. She said the teachers were cliquey, had short fuses and low energy, seemed depressed and impatient, and lacked understanding of where children were on the developmental spectrum. Some teachers still had passion but were drained. They needed to be refueled.

Libby described the bind she and many other teachers find themselves in: "When you're a teacher and you have kids of your own, you can't decompress after work. You can't just go and exercise at the gym or go to yoga. You go pick up your child at their child care program and continue until bedtime, when you are ready to collapse. There is not enough time to take care of me—other than not to work as much. Being a mom in this field has changed my capacity to do things."

Libby said that she experienced burnout during the past year. "It was hell. I think I felt burned out before I knew it consciously." Libby thought many people could not last as long as she had in this field. But Libby needed to keep plugging along to provide for household finances, her daughter's child care tuition, and other expenses. She said, "Burnout for me looks like me going home and shutting down. I do just enough to maintain the household and engage with my daughter, crying randomly, feeling unvalued and unheard, and talking to my husband solely about work."

Libby said that her school year used to start with excitement. The classrooms felt fresh, tidy, clean, and organized in the two weeks between the end of summer camp and the official start of the school-year program. "There is hope that things will get better. This year we will get it right," said Libby. But Libby found herself much more anxious at the beginning of the most recent school year. "I am doing what best practice is, but my heart is not in it." Libby explained that she wanted to figure out how she could bring joy back into her work.

Empathy in Early Childhood Education

Empathy is a character trait many early childhood professionals possess. It is the ability to understand the experiences of others and to share their emotions. Empathy is one reason teachers are so incredible at the work they do. Imagine a parent who has a week of constant arguing with a spouse. The paycheck is too small, the bills are too big, the family is about to move, and everyone in the household is overtired. This scenario would be difficult for any family. When scenarios like this play out in the lives of little children, teachers must be the steady Bettys, the calming forces, the keepers of normalcy. Teachers offer support, guidance, and resources to families. They provide empathetic ears and shoulders to cry on for families in need.

This work is invaluable, but it takes a toll on teachers. When teachers offer empathy, they open themselves up to dealing with all the heavy stuff their families bring to the program—on top of whatever personal challenges teachers may have. The emotional stew that teachers carry inside them can boil over. Sometimes it is hell to get through a day. Emotional strain contributes significantly to teacher burnout.

The toll of empathy is called compassion fatigue. Psychologist Charles Figley calls compassion fatigue "the cost of caring" (1995). Figley has done extensive research on how people in the business of caring for humans do it at a cost. Like Libby, they give generously of their bodies, minds, and souls as they work. For some teachers, vicarious trauma also takes a toll. Teachers who work in therapeutic programs take on the children's trauma and sometimes suffer themselves from depression, nightmares, and anxiety. In dealing with children who have experienced trauma and are melting down, teachers are trained to be calm, manage the crisis, and then shake it off. However, it isn't possible to shake off trauma completely. It attaches to teachers. The children's stories become a part of the teachers' stories.

This is why self-care is imperative for teachers. Teachers give so much of themselves, both physically and mentally. Constantly giving and giving can quickly lead to burnout. Self-care looks different for each person. It could be a spa day. It could be getting a coffee and drinking it in a quiet space by yourself. It could be taking a walk for some fresh air. It could be meditating for ten minutes before entering your own home after work. It could be taking a restorative yoga class. All these ideas are small but practical and effective ways to fight compassion fatigue. Figure out what works for you.

Professional development can help teachers deal with compassion fatigue too. Early childhood educators need regular in-service days, parent-teacher conference days, and staff development days. Professional development helps teachers stay up to date on research and how it relates to their work with young children. Attending a lecture or taking a class can motivate and refresh you. In-service days for planning, cleaning the classroom or playground, or setting up the classroom are essential so that teachers are not using unpaid personal time for these work tasks. Having a clean, organized classroom can also be uplifting.

Trauma-Informed Classrooms

I enjoy asking people perplexing questions that make them wrinkle their noses and think hard. In this spirit, I asked Libby about life balance. In reply, she let out a huge belly laugh that made me giggle. "Life balance?" she said. "I don't know if that is even possible with two working parents! We are organized and have routines and schedules, and it is still hard. I can't imagine what it's like for families who have one parent, three children, and no supports in place."

Libby and I talked about the population of children in her classroom. I was curious about the balance of children's needs in each room. Libby hoped to see a better balance of children with typical development and children with trauma, disabilities, and mental health problems in the classrooms at her school. She believed that an unbalanced classroom was bad for both teachers and children. She pointed out that in an unbalanced classroom, children with many needs—as well as those with fewer or more typical needs—may receive inadequate support.

Libby and I also discussed trauma-informed classrooms. A trauma-informed classroom is a place where staff recognize and understand trauma, and a place where the program policies and regulations acknowledge trauma and make efforts on every level to avoid retraumatizing children. The policies and procedures are written in a way that will help everyone. We took care to address the importance of Libby's own well-being. We read and discussed an article called "Essential Strategies for Managing Trauma in the Classroom." According to this article, "Working with individuals who have experienced a traumatic event can make someone more susceptible to secondary traumatic stress. In other words, if you're working with kids who are coping with trauma, there's a chance it could affect you too. That's why it's so important to take care of yourself—a healthy teacher is a more effective teacher." The article goes on to say that awareness is the key to managing secondary traumatic stress. It recommends regular check-ins with a small support group, regular exercise, a healthy diet, and adequate sleep (Concordia University–Portland 2018).

Reflection

- What are the differences between trauma-informed classrooms and other classrooms?

- What ideas would support a trauma-informed classroom that would benefit all the children in your program?

- How does empathy play a role in your profession?

- How can teachers who work in trauma-informed classrooms make sure that they are creating space to care for themselves and have the capacity to participate in their home lives?

- How can we make sure we are empathetic to families' needs while not taking on their problems as our own?

CHAPTER 5

Leadership

Elise's Story: In the Trenches

Elise was the director of a child care center. The center employed about 30 people (6 in leadership or supervisory positions), and served 135 children, from infants to school-age children. Elise was a fun-loving, well-educated leader who valued her staff highly. She had a master's degree in early childhood education, and she lent a hand to her team whenever possible. Whenever she came into a room, she lit it up with her smile and her voice.

Elise stepped into a classroom where the children had just returned from outdoor water play. A lot was going on, and a large pile of wet towels lay on the floor. Elise jumped in and grabbed the towels, saying, "Hey, I will go outside and hang these up for you." The teachers smiled and said, "Thanks, Elise! We appreciate that." They went back to helping the children transition to indoor play.

After a few minutes of hanging towels, Elise was met outdoors by Agnes, the program's owner and executive director. Agnes was not in direct service. She floated in and out of the classrooms. Agnes said, "Why are you hanging these up? Hanging towels is not your role. I'm concerned that your approach does not command the kind of respect you deserve. You need to start delegating."

Elise was annoyed. She always tried to support the program's staff. Elise felt that as a director, she should be in the trenches with her teachers and know what the reality was in their classrooms. Elise based her expectations on what their reality was. Elise made her staff feel that *they* were the priority—not the documentation they produced, not the standards they strove to meet. When she noticed teacher morale flagging, Elise would say, "I am going to be here to help you for the next two hours, because I can see that you are starting to burn out, and I have fresh energy."

Sometimes Elise supported others at the expense of her own needs. Elise and I chatted about her morale. She said that it was low sometimes. She believed her low morale came from having a completely disassociated owner. She mitigated this for the staff, but she couldn't do the same for herself. She felt she wasn't getting the support she needed from Agnes to keep up her own morale. Elise told me, "People cannot create effective policies and practice when they don't know the context in which they are asking people to follow through."

Be the Leader You'd Want to Follow

In early childhood education, leadership is not about being the most important and most knowledgeable person in the program. It is not about being the expert in everything and the boss of everyone. It is about humility. It is about respect for one's colleagues and respect for the children and their families. Leadership is a willingness to speak up when something is not right. Leadership is stepping up to support your teacher community and your families.

Leadership is promoting teamwork. When needs or problems arise in an early childhood program, solutions should not come down from on high. All staff involved in a situation should be involved in its solution, whether they are directors, administrators, bookkeepers, head teachers, assistant teachers, paraprofessionals, or anyone else who works in the program. Weekly tasks that benefit all staff should be shared by all staff. If everyone throws things in the garbage, everyone should have a turn taking out the garbage. For example, I work ten hours a week at a local resource and referral agency. Some employees work forty hours a week there. The staff includes an executive director, a front desk person, and many people in between. The agency has a kitchen, and everyone uses it. Everyone also takes a turn doing kitchen duty. That means emptying garbage cans a few times during the week, cleaning the sink and the microwave, and breaking down the recyclables and carrying them out to the recycling bin. These tasks may sound trivial; however, these are the sorts of tasks that wear on people and lead to low morale when they're not shared.

Leadership also means accountability. As leaders and directors, it is easy to get caught up in the quality measurement standards for environmental assessments, accreditation evaluations, and the like. However, standards aren't the only accountability tools. You can measure program quality in other ways too—ways that are authentic and based on relationships. For example, I measure the success of my family child care program in a few different ways. Of course, I have a clear idea of quality standards from an accreditation standpoint, QRIS, and regulatory compliance—and I strive for excellence in all these areas. But I also measure success using relationship-focused methods. When Monday comes, I ask myself whether I am excited to see the children and families. And are they excited to see me? Do the parents seem happy and confident about leaving their children with me? I note my longevity record with families. Are families staying in my program and referring friends? How's my record with employees? I have only one staff member. She is my sub when I need to take time off. She has been with me for more than fifteen years. While we have different approaches, she is dependable and has a lot of experience.

Accountability is essential for every person in a program—even the boss. In a for-profit program, the owner and director might be the same person. Sometimes they are different people, and the owner is the director's supervisor. In a nonprofit program, the director usually reports to a board of directors. In well-run nonprofit programs, the board of directors is active in the program fundraising, and the members have a vested interest in the success of the program. They establish bylaws and a strategic plan, and they use and revisit these regularly. The board changes over time to prevent stagnancy.

Both for-profit and nonprofit programs should have an assistant director, codirector, or other person to whom the program leader is accountable. This person must be able to shoulder responsibilities and decisions along with the program's leader. In addition, it is essential that a person in a position of power be available to take over in case something happens to the program's leader, whether it be illness or otherwise. This person should know the program well enough to be able to carry on business as usual. For family child care programs, it is equally important to have trusted backup teachers who have been introduced to families.

Some early childhood programs do 360-degree staff assessments. These are assessments that have multiple raters instead of simply a supervisor rating a subordinate. In this type of assessment, staff members answer questions, often anonymously, about their supervisor or a coworker. The questions can be about self-awareness, leadership, teamwork, and more. Many templates are available online. Whatever assessment tools are used, it's essential that leaders be assessed just as other employees in the organization are. Accountability and professional development goals need to be vital for all employees in the organization.

For family child care programs, a 360-degree assessment can be done in the form of a multifamily survey. Do parents feel their children are getting what they need in terms of curriculum, outside space and time, and so on? I believe this sort of survey is a great way to get feedback about your program, be accountable to your own philosophy and goals, and help yourself improve. Be specific in your questions, and allow room for comments. But don't ask questions you don't actually want answers to. For example, do not ask questions about tuition, late fees, hot-button issues, or policies you aren't open to changing.

Transparency is another important aspect of leadership. Sometimes directors behave as if they are secret keepers, and they give out information to staff only on a need-to-know basis. For example, a director might think, "The staff needs to know only that I am at a meeting. They don't need to know where I am, who I'm meeting with, or when I'll be back." I recently talked with a friend and fellow teacher who was frustrated about how, whenever the director left, no one was available to answer the phone at the center. The director was simply "out at a meeting." Parents, bus drivers, and potential new clients might try to call, but sadly, no one would answer the phone. Like my friend, I thought this situation was not only annoying, but also unprofessional and potentially dangerous. Emergencies and other unexpected things happen. A program must have procedures in place to get in touch with an absent director and to make decisions when the director can't be reached.

A good tool for tracking staff whereabouts is a simple in-out board with a few columns for staff names, "in," "out," "return time," and "comments," plus a movable magnetic button and an erasable marker. When employees arrive at work, they move their button to the "in" column. When they leave for appointments, they move their button to the "out" column, write the estimated time they will return in the "return time" column, and write a brief explanation in the "comments" space. When employees leave for the day, they simply move their button to the "out" column. If someone is out sick, a coworker can write that on the board. Others can look at the board and quickly see who is present, where the absent staff are, and when they'll be back.

When directors or others in leadership positions leave, they should designate someone else to be in charge. Many programs have codirectors or assistant directors for this reason. A chain of command like this increases accountability, safety, and clarity for everyone.

A final key aspect of leadership is growing new leaders. Leaders should be searching for their replacements and preparing them to lead. Leaders should watch for strengths and skills in the staff they supervise. Leaders can nurture these strengths and skills with mentoring and guidance.

A Leadership Alternative

Are there any early childhood programs in which teachers do not experience some low morale or burnout? I certainly didn't think so—not until recently.

I was two weeks away from submitting my draft of this book to my editors. I was doing an in-service on loose parts with a delightful, close-knit staff. Somewhere along the way, I commented on low morale. A staffer replied, "Nope, not here. You won't find that here." I did a double take. In my head I thought, "Say what?!" I was all but done writing the book. This new information was provocative. It challenged my beliefs about burnout. I felt compelled to find out more.

I kept my eyes and ears open while I was working with this program. I noticed several interesting things. While this staff was with me (for six hours straight), its members were 100 percent engaged. They did not check their phones; they did not text anyone; there was no beeping or ringing of any kind. The educators took ownership of their learning and were excited to apply it the following week. This focus, intentionality, and active planning were unlike other experiences I'd had leading workshops where I felt that the participants were there only physically (mentally, they were completely disconnected).

After reflecting on this unusual level of engagement, I decided to conduct an impromptu interview with the group. I had never done a group interview before, nor had I ever interviewed anyone without preplanning. Luckily for me, the educators had a lot to say about their program. The following highlights offer clues about their high morale.

The program serves children ages three to five years old. It is a parent cooperative. A parent board makes decisions for the program. The board is made up of parents who have knowledge about finance, child development, law, diversity, and so on and who are willing to volunteer. There's a finite number of spaces on the board of directors.

The staff say that having a parent board can be difficult sometimes. The board has to balance class sizes, tuition, and teacher salaries. And the board membership changes yearly, so the teachers have to get used to a new group each year. The teachers admit that advocating for themselves to a board full of parents can be hard.

The program does not have a director. Although it names a director for the sake of state regulations, no hierarchy exists among the staff. Everyone is on the same level. Being equal partners gives them freedom. Each person knows the objectives of the program and follows through. Philosophy is essential for this staff. The staff work with honesty, openness, authenticity, and agreement that they all cooperate to solve problems that arise.

The staff does acknowledge that overregulating from the state licensing agency gets them down. So does the fact that children are unable to take risks in a safe, controlled way. For example, a climbing structure at this program is safe all summer, but when winter arrives there are limitations on children using it. The cushioning material could freeze. So for six months out of the year, children are not allowed to climb on the play structure if the ground has frozen. Most teachers can make a safety assessment on a given day: if there are three inches of ice under the play structure, it's not a good idea to use it. But if it just snowed twelve inches of fluffy snow, the structure would be safe to play on. The teachers constantly struggle between allowing what they feel is reasonable, safe risk-taking play while taking the chance of getting a licensing violation, which could jeopardize the program's QRIS rating.

Veteran staffers who have been with the program for almost twenty years say that they have been able to stay and do this work because of their spouses' salaries and benefits. Even though these teachers have master's degrees, they do not make a living wage. The younger staffers who have bachelor's degrees would love to pursue higher education, but finances make that problematic.

The staff members acknowledge that their program serves an affluent population. They point out perks like having a beautiful, noninstitutional space in a lovely neighborhood, along with plenty of planning time. Compassion fatigue and vicarious trauma are not problems for them. The teachers don't take these benefits for granted. The few stresses experienced by the staff of this school simply never bog them down to the point of burnout.

● ●

Reflection

- Was Elise overstepping her boundaries?

- Do you think the teachers in Elise's program felt comfortable with her helping?

- What might Agnes's perspective be?

- How could Agnes have approached Elise differently?

- What are Elise's values as a leader?

- What do you think Agnes's values are as a leader?

- How do you think Elise should respond to Agnes?

- What does transparency feel like? What does it look like? From a teacher's perspective? From a director's perspective? From a family child care provider's perspective? From a parent's perspective?

- What is accountability? Who are you accountable to? Why?

- If you were mentoring a new leader, what are the three things you would tell this person are the most important values, ideas, or principles of leadership?

- What makes the parent cooperative story different in regard to burnout and morale?

- How might having a director or not having a director help or hinder a program?

CHAPTER 6

Professional Development

Laura's Story: An Early Educator and Higher Educator

Laura had been working for a large corporation for thirteen years when the company decided to leave the state. It invited Laura to relocate, but she had just remarried. She could not pack up and move with her new husband and three teenage daughters, who were all adjusting to life in a blended family. So Laura found a different profession—one in which she felt she could make a difference in the lives of families in her community. She met a single parent who needed child care. Her new profession started with one young infant.

Laura said that she came close to burning out three times in her early childhood education career. The first time was five months after she opened her program. She had just left a job where she'd interacted with adults all day long. Now she was taking care of one baby by herself, in the dead of winter. She felt so isolated, and she was not prepared for the toll this would take on her. Laura became very lonely. She lived in a rural community and did not know many stay-at-home parents or any other child care providers. Her first winter as a child care provider was bitterly cold and did not allow for much outdoor time with a baby.

Fortunately Laura soon found a peer support network. She heard about it through a friend. She quickly realized the value of connecting with people in her profession who could hold her up when she needed a hand. These people had open hearts, did the same work Laura did, and were willing to help her in whatever ways she needed: writing her first contract and policy booklet; helping her decline a family that could not pay her adequately and holding her when she cried about it; reminding her that she was running a business. The people in Laura's support network helped set Laura on her journey of professional development. Laura met someone running a table for a state association at a conference and was invited to the organization's annual meeting. This meeting was where Laura started really learning about all the different pathways of professional development and accreditation. This motivated her to do more.

A few years later, Laura started to feel burned out again. She was worried, unhappy, and frustrated. Laura felt as if she had no direction. Her emotions were all over the place. She could not talk herself out of the funk she was in. She decided to dive more deeply into the profession by educating herself. After attending an annual meeting of her state association, she learned of the Child Development Associate (CDA) credential and that there was an accreditation she could get for her program. She achieved her CDA credential and became accredited by the National Association for Family Child Care (NAFCC). In the early 1990s, very few family child care providers in Laura's state had achieved either of these accomplishments. For many years, Laura's program was one of only four in her state that carried NAFCC accreditation.

This accomplishment gave Laura the confidence and encouragement she needed to start helping others. After obtaining her CDA credential and NAFCC accreditation, Laura started mentoring others who were interested in following the same path. She joined the Vermont Child Care Providers Association, an affiliate of the National Association for Family Child Care, and learned a lot about association development. Over the next decade, Laura became involved with NAFCC. She attended the national conference for many years and participated in association development training. She eventually became a regional representative for NAFCC. This involvement in NAFCC gave Laura knowledge and perspective far beyond her own community. She could view early childhood issues not only on a micro level in her community and state but also on a macro level, as she met regularly with leaders all over the country via phone conferences. Laura came to realize that early childhood educators in different states faced similar challenges. For example, she noticed that the struggles around state regulations were comparable. The grass was not always greener over the state line. Laura also gained a national network of colleagues and friends who worked in a variety of settings and a variety of roles. When she had questions about local programs, she knew she could find answers somewhere in her network.

Over time Laura developed a primary clientele of children and families who were differently abled, who were experiencing risk factors, who were involved with state child protective services, or who'd had adverse childhood experiences (ACES). Laura worked closely with occupational therapists, physical therapists, speech therapists, early intervention specialists, and special education professionals in the local schools. She provided a designated specialized service program for children in foster care or those needing intensive focus on their individual needs.

Laura handled the daily upheavals with grace and generosity. She knew that she was providing a much-needed service for children and families. But meeting the extreme needs of these families was often stressful. She started to feel burned out again.

Laura reflected on this period and how it led to a huge life decision: "It was still too isolating. I thought more long-term and decided to go back to school." She did not think she would be able to keep up with her current pace of caring for children with very high needs forever. She knew that after getting her bachelor's degree, she wanted to go for a master's degree with the goal of teaching adults. This would give her an option if she decided to retire from direct service.

This was a logical next step for Laura. She had been a lifelong student with a constant yearning to know more. As a teacher, mentor, and trainer at regional, state, and national levels, she'd already been teaching about her experiences and knowledge in the field for years. So, at age fifty, Laura returned to college. She earned a bachelor's degree in human services with a focus on early childhood education. A few years later, she returned to school to get a master's degree in organizational management and leadership. She knew that securing a master's degree would enable her to go back and teach adults at a higher level. After getting her master's degree, she accepted teaching positions at two colleges. She explained, "Teaching college classes nights and weekends keeps me sane and allows me to do this with a light load of children." She could continue her family child care program but on a smaller scale. She felt that with a smaller group, she could handle the children's individual needs much better. This allowed her to feel happier and also teach at the community college. It gave her time to teach about what she loved, be with adults, and make up for the money she lost by reducing her enrollment. It saved her sanity.

Laura has remained in direct service too. Twenty-eight years after opening her program with Baby A in 1990, she sent Adult A's child off to kindergarten. The positive impact Laura has had on children and families in her community is undeniable.

Education for the Educators

In early childhood education, the demands of the field are getting more rigorous. Teachers are expected to adhere to challenging curricula and assessment systems, make sure parent-teacher conferences happen in a timely fashion, and pursue all their continuing education needs independently. Meanwhile, the pay for early educators is not going up as fast as the educational expectations of them. Most early childhood educators working outside the public school systems are making well under $30,000 per year. As education policy analyst Sara Mead points out, "Many parents, policymakers and voters still don't understand the value or complexity of preschool teachers' work and view it as merely 'babysitting.' Undervaluing historically female jobs exacerbates this perception gap." Mead goes on to say, "And the biggest challenge: How to pay for better-prepared preschool teachers (who today rank at the 2nd percentile in pay among female workers) when many parents already struggle to pay for preschool and child care" (Mead 2018).

However, the stakes are high. Research shows that children's brains are doing the most developing before age five (Center on the Developing Child at Harvard University 2007). What is more, "Early research suggested that a B.A. degree successfully identified teachers who provided high-quality care" (Institute of Medicine and the National Research Council 2012). According to education policy analyst Titilayo Tinubu Ali, "The quality of these programs is essential" (2016).

If all early childhood educators were better educated, would this reduce the number of children with failing test scores in fifth grade? Research evidence suggests that yes, it would. "High-quality, intensive ECE programs have positive effects on cognitive development, school achievement and completion, especially for low-income children in model programs designed to ameliorate poverty" (Smith 2014).

Children and adults alike build their understanding, competence, and confidence through education. Continuing education should be part of every teacher's professional development plan. Fear can be a big obstacle, though. For me that fear had to do with my history of struggling with traditional learning and test taking. I was terrified about having to take a math course. But as it turned out, going to college ended up being one of the single best investments I have ever made. I grew personally because I learned about educational, philosophical, and political perspectives I would never otherwise have known. I read books that were not only enjoyable but also left me wanting to have challenging discussions. One of my favorite required texts was *Mountains beyond Mountains: The Quest of Dr. Paul Farmer, a Man Who Would Cure the World* by Tracy Kidder. I read it on my plane ride to the World Forum on Early Childhood Education. When I finished, I was in awe of this man who was so determined to improve the health of people in poverty. At the World Forum, I then met many people who were doing similar work—advocating for women's reproductive rights, building schools in Africa, and creating safe, "normal" spaces for children experiencing catastrophes. I was moved beyond words, and I recognized that college was opening my mind and heart and helping me make connections I couldn't have made before.

If you are an early childhood educator with no college degree, facing obstacles to further education, don't despair. Laura went back to school at fifty years old. She was not alone. I went back to school at an "advanced" age too. And I discovered firsthand that education can make an enormous difference in how we teachers do our work and how well we understand human dynamics, in our perspective, and in our overall confidence. You don't have to be good at taking tests to return to school; you must simply be motivated and interested and willing to work hard. I urge you to take that first step and call your community college. I also recommend contacting the T.E.A.C.H. organization in your state to find out whether any scholarships are available to you: http://teachecnationalcenter .org/t-e-a-c-h-early-childhood.

If you are an early childhood administrator, professional development should be a regular occurrence for your staff. Seek out and offer professional development opportunities that meet individual development goals, offerings that meet the needs of the entire team, and opportunities that address the overall philosophy and objectives of the program.

Reflection

- In what ways can an ECE professional be open to lifelong learning opportunities?
- What fears does a person experience if they resist learning opportunities?
- What are the benefits of exploring a variety of learning experiences?

CHAPTER 7

Mental Health

Renee's Story: Dealing with Depression

Renee started her early childhood education career as a family child care provider in the early 1990s. For the first four years, she was dealing with an alcoholic husband, from whom she separated and then divorced. Her sister helped her out so she could go to counseling, but she still felt as if she was just existing and watching time pass her by. She said she felt depressed and unstable.

Renee realized that to keep going, she needed to take better care of her own mental health. She gave herself time and space for deep reflection, for more intensive counseling, and to attend support groups for families of alcoholics. After six months of soul searching, Renee decided to do some substitute teaching in family child care programs. This eventually turned into her business. She provided much-needed coverage for three different family child care providers so they could take a regular day off to attend meetings, expand their leadership capacity, or write a book.

For self-care, Renee took plenty of time to regularly ask herself, "What do I need?" She found that when she was feeling mentally unstable, her sister and friends could help her fill back up with what she needed.

Renee believed we could do better at teaching children coping skills to maintain mental health. Renee said, "Children need to recognize what they are feeling and be able to label their feelings. This is important so they can grow into adults who know how to handle stress in healthy ways."

Healthy Caregivers for High-Quality Care

Poor mental health is a little-discussed but important contributor to teacher burnout. Professionals in early childhood education face significant mental health challenges. The Pennsylvania Head Start Staff Wellness Survey of 2012 offers a snapshot of these challenges. This survey included 2,199 early childhood professionals in sixty-six Pennsylvania Head Start programs. The authors reported, "In our study, 24.4 percent of Head Start staff had clinically significant depressive symptoms. . . . A national study of early childhood care and education staff used the same measure and found a prevalence of 9.4 percent" (Whitaker et al. 2013). These are alarming statistics when we consider that children themselves may come from families who are already experiencing risk factors. Poor mental health among early childhood teachers adds another risk factor for these children.

Mental illnesses are common in the United States. According to the National Institute of Mental Health (NIMH), about 45 million US adults (about 18 percent of all US adults) suffer from mental illness. But only about 19 million of these people receive mental health treatment (NIMH 2017).

Mental health is serious business. It is our job as human services professionals to take care of our own mental health so that we can be whole—and so that we can provide high-quality care to young children. It is also our job to help stomp out the stigma that's still attached to mental illness and mental health treatment. Toward that end, I am open about my own experience. I understand the debilitation of mental illness. I suffer from depression. I have received treatment for depression my whole adult life.

Children cannot be joyful if the adults around them have no joy to give. If you cannot find joy, seek help. The children in your care deserve the best you that you can offer. In addition, *you* deserve to be the best you that you can be.

Finding your path to mental wellness—whether that includes counseling or medication or both—is a sign of strength, not weakness. I personally have found that I need to take medication for my depression because my emotions take a harsh roller coaster ride if I don't. I often hear people say, "I would be embarrassed to talk about my feelings with a stranger." I reply, "Not every counselor is the right fit. Find the right person, whether that means male or female or a specialist in a certain area. Ask close friends for recommendations, ask your primary care provider, or look online." Another common comment: "I would never take medication for anxiety or depression because that is a sign of weakness, and it would change me." I think to myself, "I am afraid to know what would happen if I didn't take medication over time and let my mental health deteriorate. Medication might change the way you feel, but it won't change who you are." Sometimes human brain chemistry needs balancing. Sometimes life circumstances are difficult, and talking about them helps people cope. Mental wellness means finding whatever methods help you feel well mentally all the time. If you can do that naturally, great! If you can't, that's okay too. You are not alone, and you deserve to be happy. For basic information on specific mental health issues and on mental wellness, I recommend visiting the website Helpguide.org.

● ●

Reflection

- As you reflect on mental well-being, make a list of the people who support you and whom you trust explicitly. What does their support look like? What does it feel like?

- What is the kindest thing you did for yourself today? If you didn't do anything, what will you do tomorrow?

- What can you do to focus more on your mental well-being? Be specific.

CHAPTER 8

Self-Care

Angie's Story: Art as Self-Care

Angie had a bachelor's degree in elementary education and English and a master's degree in early childhood education. She had been teaching for fifteen years at a small private school that served children from prekindergarten to sixth grade. The classes contained mixed-age groups of children. Angie had taught prekindergartners, kindergartners, first graders, second graders, third graders, and fourth graders.

Angie described the school as a "child-centered, play-based, holistic school that focuses on an emergent curriculum. We do not grade; we do not test. We do authentic assessments. We build the curriculum around the children's needs and wants; we try not to force children to have academics by a certain time and let it come to them on their own. We try to find joy in learning."

When Angie was surrounded by people who built her up, she felt invigorated and believed she could do anything. Unfortunately Angie often found herself surrounded by people who thought that early education wasn't important. Many parents, community members, and public school teachers didn't understand her learning environment and judged it harshly. Angie recalled, "I recently attended an international conference about teaching well-being to children. A woman from France asked me, 'What about the skills? Don't they need the skills?'" Angie was frustrated that even at a conference of like-minded educators, she faced judgment. "It always comes back to 'Are they going to read?'" she said. "I end up feeling undervalued."

Angie had similar experiences with families at her school. Family members seemed to believe genuinely in the school's holistic mission—at least at enrollment time—but when push came to shove, they started to worry about achievement. When Angie first started teaching there, families had not been so worried about academic skills. But over time, the academic expectations for young children had grown dramatically. More and more families asked when their children would start reading and asked Angie to send books home for reading. Families seemed to have a high level of anxiety about academic skills, and they transferred that anxiety to Angie.

Feeling continually undervalued and anxious took a toll on Angie's morale. She knew the families valued the care she gave their children, but she felt increasingly unsure that she had their respect. She was burning out.

Angie had a theory on burnout. She said that people are like candles. Their flame is their passion. It dims sometimes and burns brighter at other times. Tough times or difficult people can blow out a person's flame. But the candle is still intact. It still has wax and a wick. With effort, the flame can be rekindled.

Angie herself felt that her flame had been snuffed out. She did some soul searching. She asked herself what she needed to thrive—to relight her flame. She realized how much she was giving to everyone but herself. She decided she needed to give herself the gift of self-care.

During times of stress, Angie often found herself at the art table at her school. She followed that cue and started using watercolors to paint for pleasure. In the process, she began unpacking an incredible talent. Angie also had been occasionally doing photography. She dove deeper and turned her hobby into a business. She offered fall photo shoots for small schools and families. She used her creative eye to catch unforgettable shots, like a big brother licking his little brother. The families adored her work.

Angie's self-care involved not only indulging her creativity but also caring for her body and mind. Angie said getting a massage was an excellent method of self-care, but like most early childhood educators, she couldn't afford regular spa visits. Instead, she did things like taking long walks. She meditated regularly. She took time for daily reflection, asking herself what was taking up space in her brain. She monitored her relationships. She reminded herself that she didn't have to be friends with everyone. She instead surrounded herself with people who made her feel valuable.

Angie also surrounded herself with art, books, and music that fed her soul and helped her process her feelings. Here are a few of her favorites:

- *Daring Greatly* by Brené Brown: Angie said, "I think that in order for me to live my fullest life, I have to take risks and be vulnerable. *Daring Greatly* really reminds me to do everything I do with the openness to try, the vulnerability to fail, and the willingness to reflect on my learning and then try again."

- StoryPeople.com, a project of artist and author Brian Andreas: Angie found Andreas when she read his book of stories and drawings, *Still Mostly True*, in the mid-1990s. Angie told me, "He wrote with simplicity and clarity, sprinkled with a touch of magic. I loved that and revisited the book time and time again. Now that we live in a digital age, I follow his work on social media. When I need a reminder that life is beautiful and actually quite simple, I look to his work. I think his work also reminds me of my students. The things he writes are powerful and poignant without being too long, drawn-out, or convoluted. It's nice to get a reminder every now and then that the messy life we lead, when boiled down, is full of love, colors, and connections."

- "Still I Rise," a poem by Maya Angelou: Angie shared why she connects with Angelou. She said, "I cannot go through this life without thinking about those who came before me. Their stories, their plights, their successes. We are all so unique and yet connected. Sometimes I get weighted down by this work, the expectations on me as a wife and mother, the opinions of others. It can be too much. But when I listen to this poem, it's like a call back to myself. It reminds me to carry what I want to carry and nothing more. It reminds me to get up again and again, with pride for who I am, who I was, and who I am becoming. And I guess it also reminds me that while I can feel overwhelmed and tired, those who came before me have been through more. If they could rise, so can I."

- "I am a very emotional person. When families feel that I am doing them a disservice, I lose it. I need to cry it out, and I have songs to help me through the process." Angie's emotional playlist is as follows:

  1. "Washing of the Water" by Peter Gabriel ("I bawl my eyes out.")

  2. "I Will Follow You into the Dark" by Death Cab for Cutie ("A little more crying.")

  3. "God Only Knows" by the Beach Boys ("Then I call my husband, and he talks me down. I watch some bad TV, look up inspirational quotes, and read a good kid's book.")

A Personal Journey

Self-care is a personal journey. It goes beyond basic daily needs. It is about professional, physical, spiritual, and mental well-being. Self-care has a direct impact on all our relationships and on everything we do. Professional self-care may be taking lunch breaks and getting some fresh air, getting high-quality professional development, and participating in peer networking. Physical self-care may be getting enough sleep, going for walks, eating healthier foods, and staying home when you are sick. Spiritual self-care is about mindfulness, being present in the moment. For some people this may be meditation; for others it may be prayer. Mental self-care is about making sure that your relationships are healthy and that you surround yourself with positive people. For some people mental self-care may mean not checking their email on the weekends and making time for relaxation.

Recently a friend showed me a video of a TED Talk on "tiny habits" by Stanford University behavior scientist B. J. Fogg. In this video, Fogg describes a three-step process for changing behavior by developing small positive habits that lead toward the behavioral goal (Fogg 2013):

1. Describe the behavior you want. Be specific.

2. Come up with a way to make the behavior easy to do.

3. Identify a trigger that will prompt the behavior.

Many early childhood educators need help developing a habit of self-care. Let's say you want to exercise more. Having a goal of running a marathon may not motivate you because the goal is too lofty. Training for a marathon takes a huge amount of time and effort. However, walking to and from your mailbox is doable. You can trigger this behavior with an alert on your phone, watch, or computer. After you have achieved that tiny habit, you congratulate yourself with an "I'm awesome" and set a new, slightly more challenging goal. The next day you will walk to your neighbor's mailbox.

Research has shown that "early childhood education programs can have a positive impact on a child's success later in life. However, the annual turnover rate nationally for teachers of preschool-age children is approximately 30 percent" (University of Missouri–Columbia 2017). In other words, burnout is a huge problem in our profession. Self-care is key to preventing burnout. By caring for yourself, you become a better caregiver for children.

* *

Reflection

- Most adults lack time for self-care. We are careful to give children time and space for play. We should do the same for ourselves. How might you feel if you had some time with a set of watercolors (or some other activity you enjoy)?

- What kind of creative self-care can you make time to try? Who are the people who will do this activity with you? How long will it take, and what will you need? Set some goals for when and where this can take place.

- Create a music playlist that empowers you, motivates you, inspires you, strengthens you, soothes you, helps you process your emotions, or aids you in some other way.

CHAPTER 9

Self-Worth

Stephanie's Story: Squishy Boundaries

Stephanie had been in the field of early childhood education since
she was thirteen years old. She started out as a babysitter and then
worked as an assistant in a child care program. She'd earned her
associate's degree in early childhood education just after high school.
She'd held positions in public schools, center-based programs, and as
a nanny before she'd found where she felt she truly belonged: family
child care.

Stephanie had been running her own family child care program in
her two-bedroom apartment for nine years. Her apartment was in the
back of the complex, with access to a large yard and a beautiful wooded
area. Stephanie's home offered the best of both worlds: it was close to
the grocery store and the town's city center, as well as a natural setting
the children spent hours frolicking in. The apartment was homey,
with soft spaces and age-appropriate equipment for the infants and
toddlers Stephanie served.

Stephanie had two preadolescent sons. She was a single mom and
managed on her income alone. She did not get child support. She
worked two jobs. Her business netted $13,000 a year, and she worked
a part-time job on top of that to make ends meet. Her finances were

a constant stressor. Stephanie explained that she charged the families what she felt she should, given the spatial challenges of her home. She believed that she couldn't compete with other programs in terms of environment because her play area was small, so she had to compete on tuition.

Stephanie said that a few times she got so burned out that she wanted to close her doors for good. She had to make difficult choices that felt like she was putting her work before her family and that made her second-guess her career. Getting her boys where they needed to be was a constant challenge. She often felt overstretched. Stephanie addressed this problem by hiring an assistant. That meant a significant cut in her own pay, but it allowed her to be more present for her sons. One of her boys had some serious behavioral issues. Taking care of him through therapy took her out of her program. Stephanie felt guilty when she was not in her program and equally guilty when she had to miss an important meeting in regard to her son. Balancing home, work, and life in general was challenging—and sometimes overwhelming.

Stephanie called herself a "people pleaser." She reflected on the families she'd served in her program. Her current group was supportive and loving, but Stephanie had had very demanding families in the past. In hindsight she realized that her philosophy was not in line with theirs and that she hadn't set firm boundaries. When parents pushed her on issues that challenged her fundamental personal and professional values, she gave in. Stephanie also realized that some of her past families had taken advantage of her desire to please them. Parents would text her, asking if they had to pay her for the hours when she was out of her program. They would tell her how inconvenient her needs were for them. They showed little support for her or understanding of her situation.

Stephanie admitted that her boundaries were squishy. She said that she usually gave families what they needed unless it inconvenienced her own children. She had a fairly low opinion of her own self-worth.

Self-Worth: Teardown or Buildup

I believe that a low sense of self-worth develops equally often in early childhood professionals who work in all types of programs. A variety of causes lead to sinking self-worth. These include feeling disrespected and taken advantage of, as well as not feeling confident in the environment you have created. As Stephanie's story illustrates, constantly defending your boundaries can be exhausting. When parents, other teachers, or directors do not respect our policies and boundaries, we get worn down. Educator and psychologist Michael Formica explains, "Self-worth takes into account not only how we feel about ourselves, via identity and self-value, but also how we feel about the manner in which we interact with the world around us, through our boundary setting and management of emotions" (Formica 2008).

How Stephanie Found Self-Worth in Advocacy

Stephanie sacrificed a lot for the families in her program. In addition to money and time, she sacrificed her family space. She got rid of her dining table and skipped having a coffee table or any adult-size chairs to make space for a child-size table, a high chair, a play kitchen, a portable crib, and a creative play area. Stephanie and her boys ate dinner at the little table or sat on the living room floor. The boys couldn't watch TV when the program children were present. They had to keep their boots and jackets in their bedrooms to leave space for the other children's belongings.

Stephanie felt a lot of anxiety about her space. This anxiety chipped away at her self-worth and affected her decision making. She based her program tuition on the size of her space rather than on the high-quality care she provided; the strength of the relationships she built; and the beauty, comfort, and age-appropriateness of the space she created for infants and toddlers. She knew her tuition was well below what others were charging in her county. Her program's QRIS rating indicated the program was a high-quality program. A potential family interviewing Stephanie would expect to pay what others in the area charged. By charging so much less, Stephanie was devaluing her program not only in her own eyes but in the eyes of families. Stephanie was selfless—which might seem like a good thing—but she took it too far. She gave and gave and gave until she felt she could not give anymore. She felt completely disempowered.

I gave Stephanie a pep talk about her worth. I told her that her relationships with children and families were priceless. I explained that the cost of child care is not about the space or the equipment but about the relationships built. I also explained that it never really matters how much space or how many materials you have. It is never enough. You will always want more space or more beautiful equipment. Remember that someone, someplace is struggling to find shelter, get a meal, find child care, pay for child care, or live another day, and be thankful for what you do have. Make your space something you love. Declutter. Trade some toys and equipment with a colleague for a few months. The best way to approach each day is with optimism. Remind yourself that life will never be perfect or easy, but life is still good.

After our talk, Stephanie signed up for a professional development opportunity. It was a series of viewings and discussions of the five-part documentary *The Raising of America*. This documentary points out that the United States is one of the wealthiest countries in the world, and yet it ranks twenty-sixth in child well-being. It explains why investing in early childhood education makes good fiscal sense. It also gives a history of early childhood education in the United States. Evidence and understanding about the importance of high-quality early childhood education existed in the 1970s, and the US Congress passed a bill in 1971 providing high-quality universal child care, home visits, and other services for children from birth to age five to every family who wanted them. But President Richard Nixon vetoed this bill. The documentary challenges viewers to imagine if our country had had accessible, high-quality child care over the past four decades.

The topic sounded interesting, Stephanie knew and liked the facilitator, and this workshop would give her much-needed continuing education hours. Stephanie attended all five weeks of the workshop. The documentary was fascinating, and so were the discussions. Each week she got more fired up and came back more excited to engage with the large group. In fact, the entire group was fired up.

Meanwhile, I was watching the same documentary with a cohort of colleagues and also becoming motivated and ready to act. I felt the message of this film was critically important. I wanted more people to know why we should all be investing in young children. My now–business partner, Lisa, and I got together and talked about how energized people were. Many people needed an outlet for this energy. Stephanie was one of them.

Lisa and I developed an advocacy training called the Empowerment Project. The training focused on examining state and national policy-making systems, closing the gap between policy and practice, and helping people find their voices and use them however they saw fit, whether that was with parents or senators. People in direct service sometimes feel that policy makers just don't understand how important the work of caring for and educating young children is, and how valuable, for example, public preschool would be to our society.

Stephanie attended the inception of the Empowerment Project. Her passion was palpable. Later she shadowed me during Early Childhood Day at the Vermont state legislature. In the statehouse cafeteria, we joined other early childhood professionals to greet legislators and encourage them to attend a luncheon later that day. While I was chatting with a state representative friend, Stephanie struck up a conversation with the executive director of the Vermont Association for the Education of Young Children (VAEYC). Later, at the luncheon, Stephanie bravely offered to facilitate lunchtime conversation with a legislator at a particular table. She made a great connection with the representative and took fantastic notes.

Several weeks after that, the executive director of VAEYC got in touch with me and asked who the firecracker shadowing me at the statehouse was. She was interested in getting Stephanie on the organization's board of directors. A few months later, Stephanie was elected to the VAEYC board.

Stephanie's growth was exciting to watch. She found that she was not afraid to speak to politicians. She attended the National Association for the Education of Young Children (NAEYC) Public Policy Forum in Washington, DC, where she met Senator Patrick Leahy, Senator Bernie Sanders and his assistant, and Congressman Peter Welch's assistant. Her work on the state and national level boosted her confidence and self-worth. She'd never thought of herself as an advocate, but now she saw herself continuing on this path. She was intrigued and inspired by what she was learning and the people she was meeting.

Stephanie's involvement in early childhood education advocacy fueled her passion for the care and education of young children and helped her stay motivated in her work. It kept her going. Stephanie told me, "I didn't know anything about advocacy before. When I saw *The Raising of America* and did the Empowerment Project training with you and Lisa, it struck a chord with me. I have a fire inside of me to get children what they deserve. That is how my advocacy was born."

Stephanie's transformation reminds me of a quote from Karen Salmansohn. Salmansohn was a prominent advertising creative director before she changed careers to pursue writing. I read the following quote in her book *How to Be Happy, Dammit: A Cynic's Guide to Spiritual Happiness*: "When you realize how much you're worth, you'll stop giving people discounts" (2001). I find her writing to be exactly what I need to read every now and then. If your self-worth needs a lift, I recommend visiting her website: www.notsalmon.com.

• •

Reflection

- Do you feel that you have to sacrifice anything for your program or your job?

- Does that sacrifice help create balance or imbalance in your life?

- Does the sacrifice happen because of squishy boundaries?

- What does your advocacy journey look like?

- How can you grow as an advocate for your field?

- What strengths or attributes are you bringing to a relationship?

- What are your values? How do these contribute to your self-worth?

- What makes certain tasks more challenging or makes you feel uncomfortable?

Regulations

Heidi's Story: Finding Comfort in Change

Heidi lived in a raised ranch home, and she ran her family child care program in her lower level. It was a welcoming and warm space. She took a lot of time to think through the environment, the materials, and the activities she offered and how these would affect the behavior and the development of the children in her program. She had early interventionists, speech pathologists, developmental educators, and occupational and physical therapists coming to her home on a weekly basis.

Heidi had a clientele of families who were low- to middle-income earners and received financial assistance. She built her program to work well for these families. She told families who interviewed her, "My consistency and reliability are important for you to be able to do your job." Heidi stood behind her word—sometimes at her own expense.

Heidi had been running her child care program for twenty years. She said she felt burned out. I asked her what might have caused the burn-out. She said that state regulations were causing her stress.

Her state had recently issued revised and updated early childhood education regulations. She would have so much to add to her family handbook, not to mention more cleaning, more cushioning outside under playgrounds, more supplies to buy, more curriculum to plan, and so on. The expectations in these regulations overwhelmed Heidi. She felt they were over the top.

Bow Out, Hide Out, or Stake Out

Whenever a state revamps its regulations, the revamp makes life difficult for people affected by the regulations. The experience is no fun at all. In fact, it stinks.

Heidi's attitude was a common one. The regulations had not been rewritten in several years; it was a job that needed to be done. The state took a collaborative approach, which included stakeholders forming committees statewide to tackle the rewrite. However, the final decision-making left out many of the stakeholders. They felt frustrated and unheard, and they walked away from the process.

During any big change, there are people who choose to bow out, hide out, or stake out. In *The New Early Childhood Professional: A Step-by-Step Guide to Overcoming Goliath*, authors Valora Washington, Brenda Gadson, and Kathryn L. Amel observe that when many of us face challenges "we spend most of our time complaining or feeling victimized by them. Many of us already work long hours—or second jobs—and have precious little time. Others of us believe that we lack the skill, knowledge, strength, or community to take action" (2015, 47). We bow out. While some are bowing out, others are hiding out, focusing on "us vs. them, [feeling] discomfort with what they are being asked to do" (49). Eventually some are ready to stake out, showing a "willingness to engage in process in a deep and honest self-examination . . . to distinguish those norms and values worth preserving from those that have become antiquated and dysfunctional" (50).

Reframing

Heidi participated in a Strengthening Families Cohort. (For more information about the Strengthening Families Framework, visit https://cssp.org/young-children-their-families/strengtheningfamilies/about.) She spent a lot of time discussing and reflecting on the new regulations in small groups with other early childhood professionals. Through discussion she gained a better understanding of the hows and whys behind the regulations. Through reflection she found a lot of validation.

Studying the Strengthening Families Framework and the state regulations side by side and reframing them helped Heidi. The regulation book in its entirety was indeed overwhelming. But broken down into chunks, the regulations seemed manageable. Heidi realized that she was already doing many of the procedures exactly as detailed in the regulations—changing diapers, washing her hands, washing the floor, sanitizing tables, disinfecting doorknobs, and so on. The overall intent of the rules was to keep children safe. Like all early childhood professionals, Heidi wanted that for the children in her care.

Heidi had high standards for her program. She worked hard to meet the needs of all the children in her care with a developmentally appropriate curriculum. She was anxious about the implications of her state's new regulations on her daily activities. I asked her what she enjoyed doing with the children. She said she loved sitting on the floor playing with them. They got so engaged, and it felt terrific. I told Heidi that in the state's early learning standards, she would find a key word that appeared in different ways under each standard. This word would likely reduce her curriculum anxiety. The word was *play*. I pointed this out to remind Heidi that for children, play is learning. Children need unstructured playtime, not a highly structured curriculum. According to Kay Redfield Jamison, professor of psychiatry and behavioral science at Johns Hopkins Medical School, "Children need the freedom and the time to play. Play is not a luxury; the time spent engaged in it is not time that could be better spent in more formal educational pursuits. Play is a necessity" (Jamison 2004, 62).

The new state regulations contained some updated professional development expectations. These made Heidi anxious. They meant she would have to further her education. She did not consider herself a strong student. Heidi talked about the educational options available to her. She said she felt alternately pessimistic, realistic, and confident about them. Eventually her determination to succeed won out. Heidi decided to go to her local community college and do an assessment of prior learning (APL). In hopes of earning credit for all her years of workshops, reading, and work experience, she created a portfolio full of evidence of her life learning. She asked people to write letters to vouch for her and to support her goals. These people were specialists with degrees in Heidi's intended field of study. These people provided evidence of Heidi's knowing the information for which she sought credit. She worked tirelessly for a semester on her portfolio. The college awarded her with seventy-seven credits. Heidi would need only eight classes to earn her associate's degree in liberal arts with a focus on early childhood education. This success boosted her confidence and dramatically improved her well-being.

* *

Reflection

- If you work with a peer networking group, take some time to go over your state regulations together. Does everyone interpret the rules in the same way? Have one member take notes and email the appropriate regulating agency for clarification.

- Pool your resources by putting commonly used or useful resources into a shared file accessible to all in your networking group. One person's strength can serve another person's weakness. Determine each person's strengths, and figure out who should create forms, send emails, and create shared documents. Draw on the work of groups such as NAEYC and NAFCC and their local affiliates. Most likely, whatever you need already exists.

- Often a teacher is already doing a lot of what is listed in a "new" rule. The rule isn't really a new practice; it's just an explicit description of a previously unwritten norm. Putting these norms in writing helps inspectors know what to look for and identify compliance or noncompliance.

- Do you feel stuck amid changes happening around you? What causes you discomfort with these changes? Are these discomforts rooted in your personal temperament or in the need for programmatic changes?

CHAPTER 11

Respect

Leighanne's Story: Feeling Undervalued

Leighanne was a family child care provider who had run her own program for twenty years. She loved her work with children and families. She was well educated, had a high-quality program, and knew that she did good work.

Leighanne's main problem with her chosen profession was feeling disrespected. She believed that many people undervalued her work. She often got comments like "I wish I could stay and play all day," or "I wish I could have a naptime in the middle of the day." Some people counted heads and multiplied the count by Leighanne's tuition, then assumed the total was her take-home pay. They commented that she was "raking in the big bucks."

This feeling of disrespect festered in Leighanne until it caused a bad attitude and started affecting other parts of her life. She got cranky with her husband and her children and had a hard time snapping out of it. At the same time, she had no idea what she would do if she did not have her program. She really wanted to feel well respected.

Respect for Your Work

Over the years, I have heard many comments like the ones Leighanne heard. I assume most early childhood professionals hear similar remarks day in, day out. These comments, while probably not mean-spirited, can slowly eat away at a person.

Such remarks show that the speakers don't really understand the work we do. No one considers overhead expenses, the amount of time spent doing paperwork, shopping for supplies, nights out at networking meetings, QRIS documentation, and professional development undertaken at night and on weekends so we don't inconvenience the families we serve. As for that naptime in the middle of the day . . . well, the dishes and the documentation don't do themselves, and not everyone naps. And while we really do "play" all day, this play is interwoven with pedagogy. As we play, we are teaching children the motor, cognitive, and social-emotional skills that will carry them through a lifetime.

For example, I have a group of children who love to swing and climb all the time, and all together. I spend entire mornings and afternoons facilitating turn taking. "You can stand here. That will let Macy know you are ready for a turn. Porter, can you let Macy know you would like a turn when she is finished? Macy, did you hear Porter? He would like a turn when you are finished. Would you like me to set a timer, or do you want to let him know when you will be done?" So it goes, over and over on the swings and the ladder and the climbing structure. When communication breaks down, the children sometimes get physical, and then I use interventions and more talking. This is not just babysitting, and it's not just play. This is teaching respect, kindness, communication, and cooperation.

Disrespect is one of the top reasons early childhood educators leave the field. When people are treated with disrespect, they feel personally devalued. They feel that their work is unappreciated. The fact that this profession is mainly women-led may have something to do with its lack of prestige. According to the Center for the Study of Child Care Employment (CSCCE), "The early care and education (ECE) system in the United States is built upon a foundation of structural inequality based on gender, class, and racial inequities that are woven throughout American institutions and culture. While ECE has the potential to interrupt the consequences of these inequities, the system's current organization and financing poses multiple obstacles to educators' efforts to nurture children's optimal development and learning and implies risks to their own well-being" (CSCCE 2018).

Comments from friends and family who think early childhood teachers don't have "real" jobs can be very frustrating. We expect our loved ones to understand and appreciate our knowledge and skill. It's demoralizing when they don't. My own experience offers a good example of this. I started my family child care when my children were four months and two years old. People assumed that as soon as my kids were old enough to attend elementary school, I would go back into the "real" working world. I am not sure what people imagined I was doing during the day with children. Did they think I was not working? I would get frustrated and challenge these commenters to walk in my shoes for a day. Then I would step back and say, "Make that half a day. With no TV for your transitions and no treats as bribes. Let's see how that goes." My husband often had to tell me to calm down and take a deep breath because I would get so angry about people's comments on my work.

I have learned to laugh at such comments now. I know that it takes a very special type of person to do what I do—what all early childhood teachers do. Not everyone can love as we love, unconditionally. We can clean up vomit and diaper blowouts without gagging. We can hug children with boogers streaming down their faces, and we can celebrate their milestones with genuine pride and joy. We can solve behavior challenges like a Rubik's Cube. We can also educate people by saying, "Did you know that 80 percent of brain development happens by age three and another 10 percent by age five? That means that in the time young children spend with me, 90 percent of their brains have developed (Hunter 2017). I would say that is important work."

Whenever you interview a new family or whenever someone asks you what you do for work, use the opportunity to educate others about the work that happens in your program. Stand on your soapbox and speak out loud and clear. Own your power and your value. For example, you could start by saying, "Did you know the most valuable way for children to learn about life is through play?" If a person seems to want to know more, elaborate. Sometimes your message will fall on deaf ears, but sometimes it will sink in. Imagine the impact you could make on a parent-to-be or a grandparent who finds value in your words.

Reflection

- Do you know any early childhood professionals who have left the field due to lack of respect for their work?
- Can you think of a time when you did not feel respected or understood?
- How can you respond respectfully to people who believe your work is unimportant?

CHAPTER 12

Negativity

Nancy's Story: The Complainer

Nancy was a family child care provider who had been in the field for twenty years. She'd experienced a lot in those years and probably had a lot to offer to her peers in terms of lessons she'd learned. Unfortunately she tended to harm rather than help her peers.

Each month a group of eight to ten family child care providers took turns hosting meetings in their homes. Nancy attended these network meetings regularly. She shared a lot at the meetings. She used them as a way to get things off her chest. She complained about what wasn't working in her program. Complaining helped her feel better, but it brought a lot of negativity into the meetings. Other providers left the meetings feeling drained. They had no energy after listening to all of Nancy's issues.

We all know someone like Nancy. We attend trainings and meetings hoping to gain support, excitement, and a fresh outlook—only to have a complainer ruin our optimism and camaraderie. Negativity in one area of our life overflows into other areas.

What can we do about the gripers and moaners in our lives? Human resources consultant Susan Heathfield recommends, "Deal with genuinely negative people by spending as little time with them as possible. . . . Do not allow yourself to become drawn into negative discussions. Tell the negative coworker [that] you prefer to think about your job positively. Avoid providing a sympathetic audience for the negativity" (Heathfield 2018).

That's great advice, but it's not easy to carry out with someone who is always around. This is why it's imperative that facilitators, directors, trainers, and group leaders set ground rules for all gatherings. Make it clear that a peer network meeting is not an opportunity to bash parents who are late with payments or to bad-mouth other programs. It's an opportunity to ask for help and share wisdom. The idea is to look for solutions. If people are complaining about things that aren't working, ask, "What is working for you right now? Why do you think those things work for you?" Be an active listener and ask clarifying questions, or you may hear the same statements again and again because the complainer has not felt heard.

If you can't avoid negativity at work, avoid it elsewhere. In your private life, surround yourself with positive people who make you happy.

Laughter

I often ask the people closest to me, "What fills your soul?" Laughter fills mine. Anyone who knows me knows that I love to laugh. For me, laughing is the best balm to soothe the hurts caused by naysaying, gossip, hate, and negativity of all kinds.

Every so often I get to spend twenty-four hours at an early educator retreat with two great friends, Laura and Nicole. They get me. They do the same work I do. They have the same sense of humor as me. They love me for who I am, with all my flaws. One look or one word shared among us can unleash a snorting, bellowing, stomach-hurting, gulping-for-air torrent of laughter. That kind of laughing is just what I need to refill my bucket. After a night of uncontrollable laughter, I suddenly feel a bit more optimistic and a bit more positive.

Laughter can do this for anyone. According to the health news and information website WebMD, "Some researchers think laughter just might be the best medicine, helping you feel better and putting that spring back in your step. . . . We change physiologically when we laugh. We stretch muscles throughout our face and body, our pulse and blood pressure go up, and we breathe faster, sending more oxygen to our tissues. . . . 'The effects of laughter and exercise are very similar,' says [psychologist Steve] Wilson" (Griffin 2008).

With all the devastation in the world, it may be hard to find laughter, happiness, and humor sometimes. But it is a must for early childhood professionals. Children need joy and laughter, and the caregivers in their lives need to provide that for them.

Accentuating the Positive

When we are having trouble finding joy in our work, it might help to step back and spend a little time thinking about what we do, searching for the small joys in our job. We go through our daily lives, tending to tasks, taking care of little humans, paying bills, and cleaning. Do we take time to appreciate that we get to do those tasks? We get to take care of children who love us unconditionally. We build relationships with families in our communities. When families share their stories about their children's daily lives at home and find humor in the same frustrations we educators face, we feel connection and affection.

The work we do is not just changing diapers and hanging out with other teachers—and for those of us who are family child care providers, there's little of the latter. Our work is about building healthy relationships. As psychiatrist and child trauma expert Bruce Perry points out, "Relationships are the agents of change and the most powerful therapy is human love" (Perry and Szalavitz 2006, 230). Our work is about finding the good in every person and the positive intentions behind individual actions.

To maximize positivity, teachers, directors, and all others who work in early childhood programs must show respect to everyone with whom they interact. Respect includes open, honest dialogue with and reflective feedback from your superiors. Feedback helps us make adjustments to improve our practice. Sincere praise is a necessity too. For example, a coworker or director might say, "You have an art for getting the infants to sleep when you rock them. What is your secret?" or "I love the way you always greet the toddlers in the morning and then greet the parents. I am sure it makes them feel special." These are small, effortless ways to boost confidence. Likewise, any difficult conversation with staff or families should start with a genuine compliment.

Another key way to maximize positivity and minimize negativity is to avoid gossip. Gossip happens in most workplaces to some degree. But gossip can lead to hurt feelings, false assumptions, and unintended consequences. There is no place for gossip among professionals who work with children and families. Avoiding gossip is essential to fostering confidentiality. The drama, immaturity, and hurtful behaviors that accompany gossiping are harmful to children and families. I urge you to be the first to stand up to negative, backbiting behavior. Refuse to participate, and ask others to stop it.

If you are troubled about a situation at work or you're in conflict with a staff member or a family, take a little time to step back and think about what's happening. Taking your time allows both you and others to reflect on the situation, avoid making swift assumptions, and prepare a thoughtful response. Remember that not only you but also others may be under stress. People handle stress in diverse ways. But don't wait more than twenty-four hours to clear up a conflict. Avoiding a difficult conversation will simply encourage negative feelings to fester. Approach the issue with kindness, respect, and understanding. Try to remember that people usually have good intentions.

Be the change you'd like to see in your workplace. When a coworker starts ranting about a family who forgot their child's extra set of clothing for the fourth time, you can be the voice of optimism and understanding: "Maybe their washer is broken, or something is going on we don't know about." Perhaps you could check in with that family; you might discover that Dad dropped off every day this week while Grandma picked up, and somehow the child's clothing needs have been lost in translation. Remember—and remind your coworkers—that families are just as busy as teachers are. Families do not set out for the day scheming, "I am going to get those toddler teachers today. I am not going to bring in extra clothes. Ha ha ha!"

We early childhood educators are not well paid for the difficult and important work we do. But we are wealthy in other ways. While we advocate to improve our financial well-being, we can also be grateful for the wealth we do have, whatever that may be—a job that we love, friends who understand us, or a network of supportive colleagues. We can choose to focus on the positive instead of the negative. We can seek out a good cup of coffee, a workout, ten minutes of alone time outdoors, time with our own families in the evening, a sunset, the beach, snuggles with a baby—anything that brings us joy each day.

● ●

Reflection

- Who makes you laugh till you can't breathe?
- What characteristics do these people have that make it easy and pleasant to be with them?
- How can you surround yourself with people who make you laugh?
- How can you change the way you begin work each day in a more positive way?
- Make a list of nonmonetary wealth you possess.
- Make a bucket list of places to go and things to accomplish that you are excited about.
- Name ten things that bring you joy.

CHAPTER 13

Saying No

Ellen's Story: Learning to Say No

In 2014 I had a lot of balls in the air. I had been maintaining a five-star rating for my family child care program. This was the highest QRIS rating in Vermont. Maintaining five stars took many hours of documentation, professional development, and involvement in the community on behalf of my program. I had also been maintaining a national accreditation through the National Association for Family Child Care (NAFCC) and was serving not only on its board of directors but also as the chair of NAFCC's then-new state affiliate process, coordinating with thirteen affiliate associations across the country. On top of all that, I was involved in countless other projects. My time was completely consumed with meetings, conference calls, and mentoring peers in my community.

In July 2014 my friend Laura and I attended the NAFCC annual conference in Orlando, Florida. We both had volunteer roles at the conference and many tasks to do. I had been experiencing increasing headaches. I remember telling Laura at the conference that my peripheral vision had been growing blurry. I scheduled an eye appointment.

A week later I went to the optometrist. I told him my symptoms. In addition to the normal tests, he checked my vision fields. He confirmed that I was indeed having peripheral vision issues and some loss of vision. He said, "This could be one of two things. It could be a growth on your brain, or it could be a disease called idiopathic intracranial hypertension (IIH). Either way, you need to go immediately to the emergency room and have an MRI."

I asked, "When you say 'growth,' what exactly do you mean?"

He replied matter-of-factly, "I mean it could be a tumor of some sort." I remained calm somehow, went to the car, and called my husband. We met at the hospital at about five o'clock in the evening and spent the next eight hours there, waiting for an MRI and a specialist.

It was evident from the MRI results that I did not have a growth of any sort. I had excess cerebrospinal fluid around my brain and swelling of my optic nerve. I learned that *intracranial hypertension* means high pressure in the fluid-filled spaces surrounding the brain and spinal cord. *Idiopathic* means the cause is unknown. After several months of medication to decrease swelling, my doctor ordered another type of scan, which showed a stenosis (constriction) in a venous sinus that was likely the cause of my IIH.

In March 2015 I underwent surgery. A stent was placed in my brain to correct the stenosis. I spent one night in the hospital's intensive care unit, then went home to two weeks of no lifting. I have been great ever since. I will always have IIH, and I need to see a specialist regularly and take medication indefinitely, but I am alive and well.

This experience forced me to learn how to say no. In the months between diagnosis and treatment, I had to put my health and well-being first. The medication I took had nasty side effects. Although it effectively reduced the swelling around my brain, it also changed my taste buds, and both my speech and my memory were sluggish for a while. Terms as simple as *parking lot* did not come easily. I worked fine during the day, but by evening I was exhausted. I resigned from my NAFCC board position and freed myself from many obligations. I decided that life was too short to spend a lot of time doing things I was not passionate about or could not dedicate myself fully to. As I started to feel better, I slowly began doing more activities I had only dreamed about when I'd been overscheduled. I wrote articles for a monthly local newspaper, and I wrote two articles that appeared in *Exchange*, a magazine for early childhood educators.

While all this was happening, our state child care regulations underwent a major rewrite, resulting in a seventeen-page regulation booklet growing to over one hundred pages. It was a positive process overall, but it created a lot of work for providers. Running a child care program in Vermont had become more complicated, and the documentation was heavy. Maintaining my state five-star rating and my NAFCC accreditation was possible, but I began to wonder: was it necessary—particularly if I was trying to simplify? I chose to drop my NAFCC accreditation.

When I told people that I was no longer accredited, they were shocked. I'd always been someone who strove for excellence. I'd felt that I needed to backflip through every hoop to be the *very best* provider. But I'd begun asking myself, "Do I really have to do backflips? And how many hoops must I really jump through to prove my worthiness and the quality of my program?" Somehow I'd learned that my self-worth did not depend on saying yes to every demand. My health, my mental well-being, and time with my family were worth more than being the best at everything.

After making this change, I became more aware of relationships with families in my program. I evaluated what the families needed most from me and my program. I determined that they wanted me to love their children—to treat their children as I would treat my own. They wanted their children to be socially prepared for life after my program, and they wanted their children to be kindhearted people who made good choices. I realized that families appreciated my five-star rating, but they valued even more highly my open, honest communication and my love and concern for their children.

Prioritize What Is Most Important

A major health problem forced me to learn how to say no. But I don't recommend waiting for a health scare to learn that valuable skill. *No* is an important word that many early childhood professionals could stand to use more often. We need to say no more often, not to children but to ourselves. Caregivers tend to be people pleasers. We tend to be highly empathetic, and we take responsibility for everyone and everything around us. We put our own self-care on the back burner.

Does learning to say no mean that you stop all outside activities related to your profession? No, of course not. It means choosing activities that feed your soul. If going to trainings fuels you, then train away! If serving on a board builds leadership skills you really want, then do it. But as you do these tasks, take care not to get bogged down with them. Know when you need to take a break.

As early educators, we have a lot to do. We work long days in order to get it all done. None of us sets out intending to overextend ourselves and burn out, but before we know it, that's what happens. The tasks that once brought us joy and fed our passion become tedious and exhausting. Even before my health became an issue, I was feeling that something needed to give. My failing sight, ironically, was what brought my problem into focus for me.

Entrepreneurial consultant Alexandra Dickinson advises that we stop thinking of requests for our time as black-and-white choices. She says, "If you can't commit, you might be able to offer another solution. You may not have the bandwidth to take on the new project your boss gave you, but if you could pause work on existing tasks or delegate them to someone else, you'd be able to take it on. . . . The bottom line is, think bigger than simply 'yes' and 'no'" (Dickinson 2017).

Reflection

- What professional activities fuel you?

- Has there been a time when you had to say no?

- If so, how did it feel to say no? Were you relieved?

- Does your work hinder your health or vice versa?

- Do you have a tough time saying no?

- If so, what holds you back from saying no?

CHAPTER 14

Staff Management

Trisha's Story: Leadership Burnout

Trisha has been in early childhood education for thirty years. She worked in her program for twenty years before buying it in 2009. When she took over the program, the transition was seamless for staff and families. She had already been doing the book work and knew a lot of the financial aspects of owning a child care program, so she thought the change would not be tremendous for her either. She was wrong. The *biggest* change was for her. She realized that suddenly she had no one to share her burdens with. In all decisions, she was either the good guy or the bad guy—the buck stopped with her.

Trisha said she sometimes felt burned out. She didn't get burned out in her work by the families, children, tuition payments, or policies. Staff management was what tended to bring her down. Ensuring adequate staffing, mediating employee conflicts, and lifting staff morale took a lot of energy.

Trisha was the executive director, and she had a program director and an assistant director to help her. Both of these employees had young children, which made it difficult for them to open the program in the morning or close it in the evening. It became Trisha's job to both open and close every day of the week. She felt that she had taken on a lot of the responsibility that was once shared. She was feeling over-loaded, and knew she couldn't keep this up indefinitely.

Trisha's program was licensed for seventy children. She liked to have extra teachers on staff. This practice allowed her to give employees time off when they needed it. Without the extra staff, and since quali-fied substitutes were scarce, she would have to say no to most time-off requests. People told Trisha she was crazy for having such a high pay-roll. But she believed that this was the best way to keep her program running smoothly and her staff's morale high.

Trisha had one teacher who was extremely reliable. This teacher showed up on time all the time, and she rarely called in sick or asked for time off. She was kind, she was sweet, and she always cleaned up after lunch. However, she lacked the skills needed to work efficiently with children. This made transitions difficult for her coteachers and the children. She couldn't multitask well, and she was slow to learn new things. Three or four of the other employees complained non-stop about working with this teacher. This complaining dragged down morale. Trisha told them that others often missed work, and that this teacher always showed up and always worked hard. She was reliable, and this was a very valuable quality in an employee. (Highly educated teachers who were whizzes at multitasking did not necessarily always show up and get there on time.) The teacher had strengths and weak-nesses like everyone in the program. Trisha had found a way to focus on those strengths. Trisha believed that all her employees possessed a particular strength that was important to the program.

However, Trisha often felt as if her staff held her hostage. "I am a people person," she said. "I hate disappointing people." She won-dered if she was a bad business owner because she tried so hard to accommodate her employees. She explained, "Last school year, I asked the staff to give me their input on absolute necessities for staff-ing. I knew drop-off and pickup for their own school-age children would be a necessity for some teachers. I wanted to give them an opportunity to take turns with spouses on drop-offs and pickups. I guess I thought they would realize that every single person can't work the same shift, and that they'd use common sense and act reason-ably when signing up for shifts. But every single staff member signed up for a 7:00 a.m. to 3:00 p.m. shift. Sadly, I had to disappoint people." Trisha said she had to explain the difference between wants and needs to her staff. She assigned hours as fairly as she could, and she established a new policy for requesting time off. To her puzzlement, staff constantly requested time off on days where they could see that three other people had already made requests. Trisha wondered why teachers seemed unable or unwilling to think about coverage in scheduling. She acknowledged that this problem was her own fault. It was a result of trying to please everyone for too long and then having to reel in that impulse and get staffing under control.

Resentment, anger, and disappointment were common emotions for Trisha. She often felt that she gave a lot but was unappreciated as a leader. Trisha said that there were days when she was ready to close her doors. These days happened about once a year. She knew that she reached that point when she was trying to please everyone and stretching herself too thin. Also, she blamed "the pressure of working with fourteen people in each other's hip pockets. When one person has a difficult day, it is infectious."

Trisha had several strategies for boosting staff morale. For example, every few months she took her employees out for dinner. She also put envelopes with employees' names on the wall so people could insert nice notes in them. Every other Friday—which also happened to be payday—was massage day. Trisha arranged for a massage therapist to come in and give employees chair massages. In these small ways, she showed her understanding, appreciation, and respect for the hard work the teachers did every day.

Trisha found these morale-boosting tasks difficult when she herself was feeling burned out. To cope with this feeling, Trisha made dietary changes, sought out counseling (even though finding time for appointments was difficult), and offered a staff yoga class. In these ways, she not only took better care of herself but also took care of her staff. And she reminded herself that early childhood education was truly her passion. She said, "Even when I feel crappy, I know that I am good at what I do. That is what I go back to. This is where I've wanted to be since I was a kid. I don't know what I would do if I left the field."

Trisha encouraged teachers who were fairly new (in the field less than ten years) to understand "that what you are doing is excellent work. However, if you are burned out, do something else for a while and see if you get drawn back to children. When teachers come to me and tell me they are getting burned out, I reassign them to a different age group or classroom. That may be the change they need."

A Team Effort

Improving staff morale and enthusiasm must be a group effort. One person cannot manage the entire team's morale. That is an impossible job.

Put the focus on relationships. Continuously cultivate and strengthen relationships. Do the entire staff have to be best friends? Of course not. But they will likely spend lots of time together, and moving through the day as a team is much more enjoyable than backbiting and gossiping.

My job at a local resource and referral agency, Child Care Resource in Williston, Vermont, has taught me the value of wellness activities for the entire staff in cultivating teamwork and good physical and mental health. As an agency, we have been working better since we created a wellness committee. We've had themed potluck staff meetings, including a taco lunch, a salad day, a sandwich bar, and a yogurt bar. We've provided cut fruit to put into water to encourage more water consumption, and we've offered a yoga class at lunchtime to boost morale. (In an early childhood education program, lunchtime yoga may not be feasible, but a class at the end of the day might work.)

Your program may not have enough money to provide yoga classes or enough time for potluck lunch meetings, but there are ways to promote wellness through daily actions and words. Wellness goes far beyond food and exercise. For example, I remember having a doctor's appointment during the time I needed to be at a meeting at Child Care Resource. My supervisor approached me and said, "Your health is much more important; we can reschedule this meeting." She may not have realized the impact of that statement. It showed me that she valued me as an individual and wanted me to be healthy. If you are in early childhood education leadership, it is necessary to treat people as you would want your own family treated under similar circumstances.

Promoting wellness can mean having fun too! For example, during the holidays, the employees at Child Care Resource can opt in to a "merrymakers" activity. Participants exchange names, and then, over the course of five to seven days, they sneak around the office being merrymakers for their coworkers. They might bring their designated recipient a favorite cup of coffee or packets of hot cocoa tied with a red ribbon; hang a string of holiday lights around their desk; or decorate their office with candy canes. These inexpensive, lighthearted acts lift spirits and build cohesion in our organization. In a field full of deadlines and stress, bringing smiles to coworkers' faces can make all the difference.

Here are a few additional suggestions for boosting staff morale:

- Present a funny award for an act of kindness or a job well done. For example, at the agency where I work, two coworkers volunteered to refurnish, redecorate, and repaint the office. I bought two inexpensive succulent plants, wrapped the pots in some wrapping paper I had, printed out a tag for each that said "Feng Shui Award," and presented one to each coworker. It was silly and easy, but it made them laugh and feel appreciated.

- Keep "rainy day" jars for all employees. When you see good things happening, write down your observation for the employees involved and put it in their jars to read later on a not-so-great day.

- Go out of your way to give staff positive feedback. When you need to offer criticism or say anything that might be perceived as negative, always start with a positive comment.

- Remember that you can control only your own attitudes and actions. You can't control those of other people. So don't try to do so, and don't stress about it.

Reflection

- Think of a challenging coworker you have (or had). Think of three to five strengths that person possesses. How can (or did) these strengths help in the classroom?

- Do any of the problems or ideas in Trisha's story resonate with you?

- Could your program use any of Trisha's strategies to boost morale?

- What does wellness mean to you as an employee or leader of a program? A healthy body? A healthy mind? Happiness? Write down whatever words come to you.

- What are some small wellness goals or practices you might implement?

- How would you ensure sustainability of these practices?

- How do you think wellness lifts morale?

CHAPTER 15

Teaching Philosophy

Traci's Story: Finding Her Own Path

Traci had been in the field of early childhood education for twenty-five years. She started out assisting a neighbor who had a family child care program. Through this experience, Traci realized that she belonged in this profession. She went on to earn an associate's degree in early childhood education. She worked at a few child care centers, and then, after being a one-on-one aide in a center-based program with a differently abled child, she followed him off to kindergarten in a public school and remained with him until fifth grade.

Traci was happy in all these positions. However, she also witnessed low morale in all of her workplaces. Traci believed that there were people in every program who sucked the energy out of their coworkers. She also noticed competitiveness between classrooms and teachers. In the public school, Traci felt that the attitude toward differently abled children was quite dated. She was in the principal's office every day advocating for changes.

After her public school experience, Traci opened her own family child care program. She felt a little lost at first because the pace was completely different. There were fewer rules to follow. There was no more constant stream of time-consuming documentation to prepare for individualized education programs (IEPs). Traci journaled about how she was more present than she had ever been. She was able to notice the rain falling and watch the puddles to see ripples forming. Traci said that this aspect of her work was more enjoyable, but other aspects were more stressful. She found the business side of owning a program overwhelming and a bit bewildering. She knew she needed to find a balance between watching the rainfall and completing the practical tasks of running a sound business.

Traci had never had a clearly defined philosophy. She simply knew what she loved about some programs and what she hated about some programs. She ran her own program to include the former and avoid the latter. She had always had an enthusiastic attitude that drove her to work hard. Planning made her happy, and if someone told her she could not do something, she took it as a challenge and worked even harder to bring that plan to fruition. Somewhere along the way, she lost that enthusiasm and energy—and couldn't find it again.

One day in late 2015, she called me and confided that she wasn't feeling any joy in her work. She found herself unable to do planning for her program; it no longer made her happy. She felt unmoored. I heard the urgency in her voice and invited her to my home. Traci and I sat on the floor together, and she sobbed. She said her confidence had plummeted, and she needed help. Traci had an innate ability to provide play provocations that were thoughtful, intentional, and developmentally appropriate. But she had lost the will to create such provocations. She was desperate to rediscover the joy in working with young children. So we talked for quite some time, and I asked her many questions to help her figure out a starting point for changes in her program.

Traci decided to start by examining the different areas of her program for weaknesses and making changes in those areas. She used QRIS standards as a guide. She spent more than a year analyzing each area and changing her practice in those that she felt needed improvement. The process helped her define her values and goals.

Traci and I made a detailed list of qualities she wanted in her play-based program. She described in detail the multicultural pictures of children she wanted to have on the wall. She pulled up her Pinterest page and showed me breathtaking images of children from all over the world. Traci also shared her love for Waldorf toys. She valued their smoothness and simplicity and wanted more of them in her space. She did a self-assessment of her program space using the *Family Child Care Environment Rating Scale*. This helped her see where she needed to make changes and add materials.

Philosophy played a vital role in Traci's revamping of her program. As part of her self-assessment, she realized that none of the programs she'd worked in had a philosophy that really dovetailed with her own. In center-based programs and public schools, teachers were expected to adhere to a specific schedule. They would follow program-wide themes. There was room for minor variations but little space for individual creativity.

Traci had lots of Waldorf-, Montessori-, and Reggio-inspired ideas. She invested in what she loved to see and what she knew the children would enjoy. Each week as these changes went into effect, she and her program evolved, and Traci found joy again.

Philosophies

Early childhood education programs usually have philosophies and mission statements, likely developed when they were first established. When people form an early childhood business, they typically put their philosophical beliefs and their program goals in writing. I am always astounded when people tell me they work at a particular program but don't agree with the curriculum. I ask follow-up questions to find out more: "I am sorry to hear that you are unhappy. It must be hard when you don't see eye to eye with the program's mission. Have you ever read the program's mission statement and philosophy?" Most people say no.

If you are an early childhood educator interviewing for positions, it's imperative that you create a personal teaching philosophy that outlines your fundamental beliefs about how children grow and learn. According to the experts at the University of Minnesota's Center for Educational

Innovation (CEI), "Your teaching philosophy is a self-reflective statement of your beliefs about teaching and learning" (CEI, accessed 2018). It should also discuss how you put your beliefs into practice by including concrete examples of what you do or anticipate doing in the classroom. To begin developing your teaching philosophy, explore early childhood theorists and note the connections you do or don't feel with their theories.

From the moment you step into a potential program, your eyes should be scanning the entryway with the same scrutiny a prospective family would use. Does the program seem welcoming? Your interview is a perfect opportunity to ask questions about the program: "Can you tell me a bit more about the program philosophy?" If the program seems to be in your philosophical wheelhouse, plan a time to observe in the different classrooms to get a feel for whether the practices actually align with the program's philosophy. (Sometimes they don't.)

If you are running your own early childhood program, having a personal teaching philosophy is equally important. If you believe it, envision it. Then turn your vision into reality. Don't be afraid to evolve. If something isn't working, you can change it.

As you define and implement your teaching philosophy, take your time and be patient. The process can't happen overnight. Changes need to happen systematically. You'll need to prove the success of your practice through documentation. Intentionality, organization, and accountability are essential to creating a program that is of high quality not only on paper but also in real time, for real families, every day.

● ●

Reflection

- Do you have a personal philosophy statement? How do you believe young children should grow and learn? If you have a statement in your head, write it down. If you don't have one, use the following questions to develop your philosophy.

- Which child development theorists resonate with your beliefs about environments and about how children learn best? Here are a few resources you might explore (all by Carol Garhart Mooney): *Theories of Childhood: An Introduction to Dewey, Montessori, Erikson, Piaget, and Vygotsky*; *Theories of Attachment: An Introduction to Bowlby, Ainsworth, Gerber, Brazelton, Kennell, and Klaus*; and *Theories of Practice: Raising the Standard of Early Childhood Education*.

- What are the top five positive personal attributes you bring to your work with young children? How do those personal attributes contribute to your success or make your work more difficult to do?

- What is a perfect day in your program?

- What do you love to do that you have not had time to do recently or that you've somehow lost touch with?

CHAPTER 16

Environment

Betsy's Story: Environment as a Teacher

Betsy had run a family child care program for ten years. Her space was in the lower level of her raised ranch home. She felt fortunate to have a large room she could use primarily for her business.

Betsy said that her space worked well for her. However, she said that the children were often bored. They ran around the table constantly. They never seemed to play with some of the toys she offered.

I visited Betsy's program. I looked around and saw that she had a lot of high-quality toys and equipment. She kept many materials out to choose from. She had created defined play spaces, but there was too much stuff in each space.

We walked around the space together and talked about what the children were most interested in within each area. I asked her what she thought would happen if she boxed up and put away half of the materials that were out. Betsy looked at me quizzically, not sure if I was serious. I said, "Maybe rotating some of the great stuff you have would rekindle the children's interest." I explained my idea.

Betsy agreed to try my suggestion. Together we removed about half the materials. We reduced the number of dolls and accessories, boxed up half the kitchen utensils, and set up a block center away from foot traffic. We created a new area specifically for quiet time—a soft, comfortable space for reading books. We moved the table to a corner, making it harder for children to run around the table. We also removed half the clothes that were in a dress-up basket and hung the remaining ones on some hooks.

The children returned the following Monday. Betsy reported that they became engaged immediately. They knew exactly what to do and where to go. More imaginative play happened. Even she felt happier in the reorganized space.

Classroom Refresher

Walking into my kitchen or the room where I do my writing and seeing clean, open spaces feels great. A clean counter or a clear desk, all wiped off and sparkly, makes me happy. Unfortunately this isn't usually the state of my home. Most of the time, the surfaces around my house contain clutter piles—piles in the cubbies, on the island in the kitchen, next to my chair in the living room, and on the dining room table. These piles grow and become thorns in my side.

I have to deal with this clutter about once a month in order to feel that I really have a handle on my home life. I need to do this with my child care space too. Through the nonstop activity of me and the children, things get out of place. Sometimes they fall behind the bookcase or toy shelf. I have to make an effort to put the space back together, or it becomes chaotic and begins to affect our emotions and our ability to function.

Psychologist Sherrie Bourg Carter (2012) explains, "Clutter can play a significant role in how we feel about our homes, our workplaces, and ourselves. Messy homes and work spaces leave us feeling anxious, helpless, and overwhelmed."

This is just as true for teachers specifically as it is in general. A study by teacher educators Glen Earthman and Linda Lemasters showed that teachers who worked in conditions they considered unsatisfactory tended to question whether they would stay in their profession. According to their report, "Any aspect of the physical environment that distracts teachers from the main emphasis of instructional activities influences the degree of their effectiveness. When heat, cold, lighting, and acoustics, for instance, work against the efforts of a teacher in the classroom, some compromise or accommodation must be made in the work of the teacher. Usually, such compromises result in more intense effort on the part of the teacher to do those things that are necessary to properly teach students. . . . Negative perceptions and attitudes about school facilities carried over a period of years eventually leads to low morale and burnout, even among the most undaunted of teachers" (Earthman and Lemasters 2009, 323–34).

Is your space pleasing to you? If not, it probably affects your mood each day. In addition, imagine how it must feel for children and their families day after day. Since you and the children may be spending ten or more hours each day in your space, make it a place that brings you pleasure.

Does your space reflect your values? How do you visually communicate your values in your space? Diversity, inclusion, music, art, family, friendship—whatever your values are, let them shine for people to see. When they see your space, they'll learn a little about who you are.

Are you a "collector of all things"? Many educators—especially early childhood teachers—are. As an early educator myself, I know how easy it is to collect too much stuff. I notice items at thrift stores or things friends are getting rid of, and I see value in them for loose parts play. We teachers are famous for saying, "I may need that for something, sometime." Soon we have a lot of stuff lying around.

Having an adequate supply of materials for play and learning is a good thing, but it's important to recognize when "enough" becomes "too much." When an environment becomes cluttered, its inhabitants start disliking the space. Grumpy feelings develop; problematic behaviors erupt; messes get harder to clean up. If you notice these signs, it is time to purge. Stop wondering when that item you salvaged three years ago may come in handy. Think about the amount of space you have and what is sensible to keep. Indoors, start by getting rid of damaged, chipped, cracked, or broken toys and ripped doll clothing. Outdoors, cull broken buckets and shovels and cracked toys; clean out flower beds; and drain any standing water. Get rid of items that the children don't seem to enjoy or haven't used in a while. Once you've done this challenging work and you see the full bags and boxes leaving your space, you'll realize how crammed it was and how much better it now feels.

Reorganize what remains. A space meant for children's play and learning must be aesthetically pleasing and not overstimulating—to both children and adults. Spending upward of ten hours a day in the same space with several other humans can be stressful. A space that is calm, pleasant, and organized can mitigate stress. When you walk into your space, do you feel good? You want to feel as if you have arrived in one of your favorite places. To create a homey environment for the adults, post an inspirational quote on a small poster and hang framed photos of loved ones.

Create a "yes" environment. This is an environment that meets the individual needs of the children in the group and has developmentally appropriate activities available to choose from. It is safeguarded so children can play uninhibitedly.

Get on the children's level and look around to see what they see. That will help you see the environment from their perspective and give you ideas for how to better equip the space for small people. For example, is anything hung at the children's eye level? Many people tell me they don't hang artwork low because children will tear it off the wall. My response? Let them. Noticing and exploring beautiful things with all the senses is an important part of child development. To protect low-hanging artwork, frame a piece of plexiglass on three sides so you can easily slide artwork into it and out of it. Also, you could hang some artwork up high and some down low.

Change is good for the children and adults in an early childhood space. Rotating and refreshing toys and other materials creates excitement. Rediscovery and new learning happen when the environment changes. (See appendix C.)

Reflection

- Does your environment reflect your philosophy?

- How long have you had the same room arrangement or paint color?

- Does your environment need a facelift?

- Does the space you spend so much time in make you happy?

- How do you feel when you walk into your program space after a long weekend?

- If you feel overwhelmed by clutter, this could be dragging down your mood and energy. Make a list of where the piles of clutter are and prioritize what you should tackle first. What is in each pile? Do you need to keep it? Is it information that's now available on the internet?

- Does your space meet the needs of the children in the program?

- Does your space meet the needs of the teachers?

- If not, what changes can you easily make to better meet the needs of children and adults?

- Consider creating a wish list of items you need and posting it on the classroom door. (See appendix A.)

CHAPTER 17

Peer Networking and Mentoring

Beth's Story: Reaching Out

Beth had been in the early childhood education field for more than twenty years. She ran a center-based program for a few years before realizing that her heart was really in smaller programming. She built a beautiful space in her childhood home, which she and her husband bought from her parents. The program flourished, and Beth became highly respected in the community.

Beth's husband was in the US military. She wholeheartedly supported his career, but she said it brought her a great deal of anxiety. She noted that military families faced a higher possibility of burnout. "Military life has been a strong and positive experience overall," she said, "but it is challenging. We deal with several weeks a year of annual training on top of months-long deployments. When your spouse is away, all the family responsibilities fall on the one left behind. These times add so many stressors to our everyday lives, and sometimes these stressors spill into our professional lives. For family child care providers, the children's families become not only professional but also personal connections. They are in our homes every day. They hear, see, and sense when life is challenging for us and we are struggling."

Beth's anxiety was persistent. She said she managed it either by laughing it off or by having insomnia. She struggled to get enough sleep most nights. She took measures to combat her anxiety and fatigue by gradually moving her program's closing time earlier, working out in the morning, and sometimes going to spinning classes at night. She also set aside time to meditate and journal. While these measures helped, she still could not shake off the anxious feeling in the pit of her stomach each day.

Beth eventually realized that her self-care measures were not enough. She needed to reach out and ask for help from others too. She explained, "I think we all reach that burnout point sooner or later. For some of us it might happen several times during a career. I think it's necessary to have a peer group and to reach out to your peers when you're feeling depleted. I need to work on asking for help and guidance more often.

"I think having a mentor is key," Beth continued. "My mentor has helped me obtain a level of professional development I night not have achieved alone. She is always available. She listens and offers advice and guidance. She brings me back to reality when life is overwhelming and I am about to crash and burn. Mentors may not have all the answers, but they understand us and want to see us succeed. This career can be very isolating, with minimal adult interactions. Utilize the people in your life who value and understand you."

Beth learned to identify her symptoms of low morale and to act on them. She said, "It feels like no motivation, no drive, no enthusiasm. My tank is empty. I'm feeling overworked, overwhelmed, and underappreciated. I've learned that it is important to have people around me who can fill me up when I'm feeling depleted—who understand how my brain works and who value my career path."

The Importance of Support

Peer support is one of my go-to self-care techniques when I am feeling fried. Often what I need most is someone who understands the work I do. I believe that my peers have helped me as much as I have helped them.

Research evidence suggests that peer support is crucial to teacher retention. A large review of studies on teacher retention published from 1980 to 2003 conducted by the Rand Corporation found that "schools that provided mentoring and induction programs, particularly those related to collegial support, had lower rates of turnover among beginning teachers" (Guarino et al. 2004, 62). One study in this review identified that "the strongest positive factors were having a mentor in the same field, having common planning time with other teachers in the same subject, having regularly scheduled collaboration with other teachers, and being part of an external network of teachers. . . . Turnover was less likely the greater the number of supports" (219).

But peer support isn't just for beginning teachers. According to researchers Marcy Whitebook and Dan Bellm, "Historically, mentoring has been thought of as a strategy to support new teachers, often within the context of their pursuit of higher education, but mentoring now takes place in a wider range of settings, with variations in mentoring goals and mentor-protégé relationships. Most mentoring programs today are designed in the service of quality improvement and are supported by a blend of public and philanthropic dollars" (Whitebook and Bellm 2014).

It's imperative to surround yourself with positive individuals who love you and care about your well-being. Reach out to a peer or a mentor when you are having a difficult day and you know you need a lifeline. That person will understand what you are going through. For example, when Vermont's weather has been below zero and I have been stuck indoors with young children for days, I know I can call on a local friend who also does child care, and she will understand my struggles.

Networking with peers at conferences and local meetings or volunteering through a professional association can bring an early childhood teacher a much-needed lift. When you meet with like-minded people, you can share challenges and celebrations and offer support in a way that non-teachers may not understand. Seek out an early childhood educator union, local association, or state network in your area. Depending on your state's regulations, you may earn professional development credit by attending such meetings. Even if you don't, simply having time with a roomful of your peers can be uplifting.

Here are some tips for effective peer networking groups:

- When you are discussing problems, always look for solutions. Do not let meetings turn into sessions full of complaining about what can't be done. Look for what you *can* do to fix a situation.
- Welcome people from all programs. Do not draw lines between center-based and family child care programs. We are all doing the same work. We all want the best for children and families. We all can learn from one another.
- As a group, identify topics, conversations, book discussions, self-care activities, or other desired activities. Plan them for the entire calendar year so that people can choose in advance which meetings to attend. Time is precious.
- Take turns bringing a snack to meetings or hosting meetings in different homes or other locations (centers, libraries, coffee shops, and so on).
- Create a private Facebook page where your group can discuss issues that are important to them outside of scheduled meetings. This page can also be used to share meeting times and locations, as well as other important announcements.
- Create guidelines regarding confidentiality and respect for the network and Facebook page.

If you are looking for discussion topics, here are some children's books that carry great messages for peer networking groups:

- *The Day the Crayons Quit* by Drew Daywalt
- *Miss Tizzy* by Libba Moore Gray
- *Miss Rumphius* by Barbara Cooney
- *Swimmy* by Leo Lionni
- *The Crown on Your Head* by Nancy Tillman
- *Beautiful Oops!* by Barney Saltzberg
- *The Three Questions* by Jon J. Muth

And here are two books to bring positivity and optimism to the classroom:

- *Life Is Good: The Book* by Bert and John Jacobs
- *The Power of Positive Thinking* by Norman Vincent Peale

In addition to having a peer network, having a mentor—either within or outside your program—can help you keep goals within sight and be accountable to your goals. A mentor is often your biggest cheerleader. I had a mentor early on in my professional career, and she helped me become a leader and create the highest-quality program I could. She had a wealth of information at her fingertips, and I wanted to soak up as much of that information as I could from her. Find someone who has a vast knowledge of the early childhood profession, an open mind, and good listening skills.

● ●

Reflection

- How can you use your peers to keep yourself accountable?
- How can coworkers help you feel supported?
- What does being supported feel like to you?
- If you find yourself feeling unsupported at work, where else can you look?
- Can you identify a colleague who might be a good mentor for you?

CHAPTER 18

Empowerment

The early childhood education profession is experiencing a quiet crisis. People who are talented and passionate about this work keep leaving the field. For all the reasons described in this book's earlier chapters (and more), their morale has plummeted.

The word *morale* has several definitions in the *Merriam-Webster Dictionary* (2018), but two of them are especially relevant to the work of early childhood care and education:

1. The mental and emotional condition (as of enthusiasm, confidence, or loyalty) of an individual or group with regard to the function or tasks at hand

2. A sense of common purpose with respect to a group

Advocacy

Let's start with the first definition. People get stuck. Frustration and disappointment with various aspects of their work build up inside them. They feel helpless and lose their spark. It is hard to relight that fire.

Getting angry about the problems we see can relight our fire. I've seen this happen many times. My friend and colleague Lisa Guerrero and I both viewed the 2015 documentary series *The Raising of America: Early Childhood and the Future of Our Nation*. (For more information on this film, see page 58.) Lisa facilitated a five-part viewing and discussion with a group of early childhood educators, and I participated in a similar viewing and discussion group with a Strengthening Families Cohort.

What happened following each viewing was extraordinary. People got angry that the United States is the richest country in the world yet is rated twenty-sixth for child well-being. Despite clear evidence to support investment in young children, we still don't do nearly enough. People asked questions. "If the United States is the richest country in the world," they wondered, "how come we can't get this right?" They had strong, informed opinions about what young children, families, and early educators need but aren't getting. They wanted to see a hefty investment in the early childhood system—not only to raise the quality of programs through educating the workforce but also to help families who cannot afford quality programs and do not qualify for subsidies. Lisa and I recognized this anger as an opportunity to arm them with knowledge and understanding about the systems (within our programs, local councils, state governments, and the federal government) that create policy affecting early educators, children, and families. Thus armed, they could *be* the change they wanted to see.

A business called Positive Spin, LLC, was born from these conversations. Through Positive Spin, Lisa and I wanted to help early childhood educators—and anyone else who cares about young children and their families—feel empowered to join the work of early childhood systems change in the United States. Inspired by the work of early childhood scholars Valora Washington and Stacie Goffin, Lisa and I dug deeply into our small state's early childhood system. For information, advice, and inspiration, we used Washington and Goffin's book *Ready or Not: Leadership Choices in Early Care and Education*, as well as *The New Early Childhood Professional: A Step-by-Step Guide to Overcoming Goliath*, a book by Washington, Brenda Gadson, and Kathryn Amel. These authors understand the plight of the early childhood education field. Professionals in the field need to find common ground, become better organized, and cultivate leaders.

As Positive Spin, Lisa and I developed a five-part advocacy training series called the Empowerment Project in 2016. The training focused on examining systems and helping people get involved in change however they saw fit. Participants in this series told us they were tired, underpaid, feeling ready to leave the field, frustrated by the lack of communication between policy makers and direct service providers, and so much more. Decisions were being made and QRIS standards created with no input from the workforce.

After completing exercises that helped them explore assumptions, define problems, and suggest solutions, the group identified some areas on which to focus their efforts. Participants wanted to bring attention to the lack of respect for early childhood education, the need to maximize resources, and the tension caused by new licensing regulations. We then invited a panel of policy and systems folks (representatives from our state's child development division, our local NAEYC affiliate, and local coalitions) to listen to participants' ideas, questions, proposed solutions, and potential projects. Before the panel event, the group learned and practiced constructive dialogue skills so that a productive conversation could happen. Its purpose was not to debate but to learn and understand how to move forward.

Early childhood educators Paula and Trisha were participants in the first Empowerment Project. They suggested to the panel the need for an action plan that would bring wider attention to legislative issues. They asked about a rally. This idea became a reality nine months later. Paula and Trisha planned and carried out a rally on Vermont's Early Childhood Legislative Day. At the rally, a parent spoke about her challenge to pay for child care. A director spoke about the challenges of finding qualified teachers and the importance of legislative support of the TEACH grant program that provides scholarships for early childhood educators. A family child care provider spoke about fair compensation. This rally has become an annual event.

A few months later, an early childhood educator approached Lisa and me at a VAEYC conference. She told us that she'd shown up at the first session of the Empowerment Project thinking that she would likely not attend the following four sessions, since she'd been planning to leave the field. But the first session inspired her, and she showed up to all five. The Empowerment Project helped her find a greater purpose, and she is back in school, finishing her bachelor's degree in early childhood education. Another participant met the president of the VAEYC board of directors during the series and shortly thereafter joined the board. A few of the participants who were quiet during most of the series surprised us by asking many questions of the panelists. Since then these participants have become actively involved and vocal about their concerns.

By encouraging people to step outside their comfort zones, the Empowerment Project has catalyzed a morale change in early childhood professionals in our area. Participants have gotten involved in advocacy by joining state association boards, writing op-ed letters about legislative issues, and contacting representatives and senators, as well as having difficult conversations with directors and families. A friend of mine who participated in the Empowerment Project is now leading a peer network. After attending a statewide meeting for the first time, she remarked, "These meetings help me realize that my work is important and there really are people out there that care about what we do." She felt valued. Talking about the hard work we do and advocating for children can make us *feel* powerful and help us *be* powerful.

In our advocacy trainings, Lisa and I often use this maxim: "The magic happens outside your comfort zone." Paula was recognized as a Vermont Early Childhood Superhero because of her work on the rally. When we congratulated her, she said, "None of this would have even been on my radar if you hadn't shown me where the magic was hiding all this time." She'd been empowered by stepping out of her own comfort zone.

Like Paula, I was not always an advocate. Advocacy didn't come naturally to me. It has taken me years to learn about the systems and factors that affect early childhood care and education. (And I am still learning about these.) It took me years of doing the work I do each day with children and families before I began to spot where the system is failing. It has taken me years of asking questions, even when I felt silly asking them. Over time I have learned that sometimes I need to go out on a limb and expose myself to critical feedback or a differing opinion. Each time I do this and feel heard, it gives me a bit more courage, and I stand taller the next time.

Through this experience, I have found that being an advocate in my profession is one of the single best ways to refuel when I am burning out. If you have a passion for the work you do, that is all you need to get started. I encourage you to show your passion through advocacy work. Take a chance. Speak up. Who knows—you may even find your next calling as a lobbyist or politician! When you speak up, you are setting an example for your own children and the children and families in your care. They are watching you and are inspired by your courage. Your voice may shake, but step forward anyway.

A Sense of Purpose

Now let's take a look at the second definition of *morale*: "a sense of common purpose with respect to a group." All people, regardless of the work they do, need a sense of purpose. Just showing up day in and day out does not sustain morale. People need motivation to sustain their work.

Motivation, in turn, requires goal setting in the form of a professional development plan. Often people write professional development plans because their employers or state regulations require them, and they do the task quickly to check it off a list. In such cases, the goals people set may not have any personal meaning or practical purpose. Often the plan is not revisited until a year later, when it needs to be updated. At that point, the plan is surprisingly unfamiliar.

It is helpful to have a director, head teacher, coworker, or mentor with whom you can talk about goals and brainstorm an efficient, effective path toward achieving them. Accountability in your goals is important to your professional growth and your ability to stay passionate about your work. Countless times I have sat with individuals whom I mentor, helping them write professional development plans. (See appendix B.)

I try to guide people to be intentional and thoughtful about their goals. Together we set professionally meaningful goals. Then we create a map with detailed actions and checkpoints. The plan is meant to be revisited throughout the year, so when the individual is required to update it, the old plan contains lots of notes and dates showing the person's challenges and accomplishments.

Personal goals are just as important as professional goals. Think about setting personal goals while you are setting professional ones. Empower yourself!

● ●

Reflection

- Does your state have an early childhood legislative day?
- What groups advocate for children in your state?
- Research which local organizations do advocacy at a state level for issues such as the following:

      financial assistance
      rights of child care providers
      public preschool
      regulations
      hunger
      homelessness
      child and adult food programs

- Who is someone you believe can keep you accountable?
- Does your state or employer require you to do professional development plans or self-assessments?
- Will you feel more motivated if you set small goals or large goals?

CHAPTER 19

Playfulness

Several years ago a group of people entered my world and changed my thinking about not only my work but my entire life. They made me into an optimistic thinker, believer, and doer. These people were from the Life Is Good Kids Foundation, which partners with child-serving organizations to positively influence the quality of care delivered to the most vulnerable children. Its Playmaker Program offers retreats, tools, and coaching to professionals in schools, hospitals, social service agencies, and enrichment programs to help children overcome trauma associated with violence, poverty, and serious illness (Life Is Good Company, accessed 2018).

I participated in a Life Is Good playmaker training. A playmaker is someone who develops optimism in children who desperately need it. In this chapter, I want to share a few ideas I learned from this training. I hope these ideas will create enthusiasm, spark some joy in the work of early childhood educators, and change the culture of our workplaces.

In my playmaker training, I learned how important it is for each person who works with children to have a personal playfulness plan. The caretakers need to care for themselves as well the children. In my experience, many of us are terrible at this. We can start practicing self-care by asking ourselves a couple of simple questions: "What feeds my heart and soul?

What fills me up with joy?" (For me, the answer is by watching my children play lacrosse, sitting by the lake drinking coffee, and dancing to live music.) After we answer those questions, we need to make time to do the activities that feed us and keep us balanced. It is easy to forget joy when morale is low. We need constant reminders. In search of reminders, my group at the playmaker training milled about looking at hundreds of photos, looking for images that spoke to us. The trainers then created a pictorial play plan using our selections. I keep this collage as my wallpaper on my phone and tablet so I remember that I need joy—and remember what brings me joy.

I had the privilege and pleasure of forming some lasting relationships in the Life Is Good family. One of my new connections was with a woman named Carly McPartland, an elementary school teacher from Pennsylvania. I asked Carly to share her story. (For details on the games described in Carly's story and elsewhere in this chapter, visit the "Games and Activities" page at the Life Is Good website: https://content.lifeisgood.com/kidsfoundation/resourcehub/play-2.)

Carly's Story: The Power of Being a Playmaker

It's usually the rubber chicken that gives me away. It could be the hundreds of brightly colored plastic cups stacked on a low shelf. Maybe it is the parachute draped over my shoulders like a royal robe as I meander throughout the classroom. My style of mastering standards while making memories is a little unusual.

I didn't start out as this kind of teacher. A transformation within me led to this effervescent classroom environment. From this experience, I reemerged a more playful, present, and passionate person.

In the spring of 2013, I was approaching the end of two long, hard years of teaching. I was feeling burned out and broken down. My first two years as an educator had me wondering if teaching was meant to feel so draining, unfulfilling, and overwhelming. It pained me to admit it, but I believed that I needed to move on from my position and seek out different teaching experiences.

As I searched for a new job, I contacted a friend who worked for the Life Is Good Company. I learned about the Life Is Good playmakers. These superheroes of healing provide training to individuals working with children who have been traumatized by serious illness, violence, or poverty. In my brief time teaching, I had already had numerous students who fit that description. I knew I could benefit from the Playmaker Program. I could bring the lessons I would learn to students who really needed them.

That May I traveled to Boston to begin my playmaker journey. I knew the trip would teach me valuable techniques to support my students' growth and development. What I had not predicted was the rejuvenating experience of connecting with kindred spirits whose mission it was to help kids live playful, joyful, love-filled lives, regardless of circumstances.

When I arrived in Boston, I walked into a hotel ballroom to discover a circle of chairs filled with smiling teachers, counselors, child life specialists, and pediatric medical personnel. Right from the start, we spent our day playing. As part of a game called Newsball, we shared our news before the whole group and received the reactions we chose, as well as emoted different reactions for others. We connected to what brought us joy through another game called Cool Breeze Blows. We played with an enormous parachute, fueled by teamwork and adventurous hearts. In a game called Wrecking Ball, we stacked plastic cups and decided whether we wanted to knock them down or keep them standing. This game, like others in the Playmaker Program, aims to give children control within their own lives at times when they feel helpless. As we played these games, we learned why this kind of engagement matters. All children, especially those facing serious difficulties, deserve to feel like kids. Throughout the day, I found myself laughing and smiling more than I had in months. I felt free just to be myself.

I jumped at the chance to become a certified playmaker four weeks later. During two more action-packed days of training, I did many activities meant to bring participants joy, social connection, internal control, and active engagement. I learned the power of creativity as we evolved a simple game of tag into truly immersive experiences with the use of imagination. We climbed chairs in an effort to win a team-building game of Musical Shares, and we lost track of competition as we played a game called I Don't Know Whose Team I'm On Dodgeball. We created individual playfulness plans to keep the fires of innovation and playful spirits burning in our personal and professional lives. I left with a heart full of joy, a head full of ideas, and a duffel bag full of materials to bring healing playfulness to my students.

Returning to my classroom the following fall, I was eager to share what I had learned with my new students. I started our year off with the same circle of chairs I'd found at the start of my playmaker journey. I was determined to create a welcoming space for all students and all emotions.

What we created as a class was nothing short of miraculous. The students instinctively followed my playful example. Before beginning any endeavor, we asked ourselves, "Is it safe? Is it fun?" It was common to see our class mascot, a rubber chicken named Chuck the Chicken, fly across the room as we played a game called Sparkle. We played Musical Shares, setting a classroom record of fitting twenty-four students on five chairs. We took the beach ball in our hands and played Newsball. We passed the ball around the room, and we each told our classmates what we felt most needed to be heard—and how we wished our news to be received. Following the ball as it made its way from table to table, we also followed the roller coaster of emotions. In these moments, we learned from one another, about one another, in front of one another. Secrets became a thing of the past, and bullying dared not cross our threshold. We even kept a classroom journal where students could jot down game ideas of their own, eventually teaching the game to the whole class.

Playmaking isn't just a classroom management technique. It is a lifestyle, a shift in perspective. My students and I are equals who deserve to feel safe and joyful. We are each, in our unique way, enough. We use these principles to guide us through our connected learning journey. This change in perspective has been critical in helping me move forward as a teacher and as a human being.

As teachers, we are often asked to overanalyze, overplan, and over-whelm our systems. When we're living and working this way, being present means a check mark in an attendance box, not being mentally present. Through my experiences inside and outside the classroom, before and after my playmaker training, I learned how crucial mindfulness and presence can be. What we do not have as educators, we cannot give to our students. We know that is true of knowledge, skills, and wisdom. But what about presence, imagination, and joy? By cultivating my playfulness, joy, and presence, I have become a happier, healthier individual and a better teacher.

Playfulness drew me back from the brink of burnout. What is more, I learned that making the mundane tasks enjoyable in all aspects of my life can change the mood of an entire day, week, month, or year. I doodle while waiting at the DMV; I try to make a three-point shot into the laundry basket; I run dishwashing time trials during my evening chores. When I begin to feel stress and tension inundating my system, I seek out what makes me joyful—whether it is reading, attending a concert, visiting with friends, or gratitude journaling—and allow myself the time to engage fully in this joy.

The biggest change in my life has been the reignited passion and positivity I feel toward teaching. I no longer cry for my students as they leave my classroom at the end of the year, worrying about their uncertain futures or unpredicted struggles. I know I have helped them develop optimism and joy, and they carry those critical tools with them. As they walk away from me, I see the leaders of tomorrow—passionate, purposeful, and positive human beings who can lead the way for others.

Goodification

You won't find *goodification* in the dictionary. The team at the Life Is Good Kids Foundation made up this word. Goodification is a bit of magic we can perform when we have to do tasks we are not so fond of doing. For Carly, those tasks are laundry and dishes. She goodifies them, or finds ways to make these tasks enjoyable. Playmaker trainer Emily Saul dislikes taking out the garbage from her apartment. It is quite a task. She has to carry the trash down a few flights of stairs and walk across the parking lot to the dumpster. She decided to make this task she dislikes into a game. She started timing herself when she takes out the trash. She runs down the stairs, runs to the dumpster, and runs back up the stairs, trying to beat her fastest time. Now she says, "I *get to* take out the trash," instead of, "I *have to* take out the trash."

I went home after the training and decided that I could play this goodification game. I dislike unloading the dishwasher every morning. So I made up a dishwasher game, and it goes like this: I turn on the coffeemaker, and it needs to warm up. I try to empty the top dishwasher rack by the time the coffeemaker is warmed up. Then I set it to brew a large cup for my travel mug. I race to unload the silverware while the coffee brews. Lastly, I brew another small cup to finish filling my mug. Then I unload the bottom rack as fast as I can. With this game, I've turned "I *have to* empty the dishwasher" into "I *get to* empty the dishwasher."

Turning a *have to* into a *get to* is a game changer. Anything can be goodified. We can goodify mundane tasks, staff meetings, you name it. We can even goodify those oh-so-common but oh-so-grating early childhood behaviors, such as name-calling, hitting, hair pulling, and pushing. Tweaking your approach to these behaviors can disrupt the negative flow they create in your classroom.

For example, being called a "poopy butt" and "poopy head" by the children in my care for days on end was wearing me down. I ignored it; I acknowledged feelings; I talked to the children about it. They just kept doing it. After spending a weekend away from the children, I came back ready to goodify. I was going to goodify all the things!

The name-calling began again at cleanup time. I asked, "What are some other names you can call me—names that will make me feel good?" I suggested, "You can call me Princess Ellen. You can call me smart and lovely. You can call me honey. You can call me Ella, or what my mom used to call me: Ella Belle."

A four-year-old chimed in, "We could call you mermaid or bird."

I replied, "Ooh, what kind of bird could you call me?" The bird suggestions went on for quite some time.

Later that day I heard "poopy butt" again. I calmly said, "What are some other names you can call me—names that I like so much better?"

The children as a group started rattling off the earlier suggestions: "Ellen, mermaid, princess, birdie. . . ."

I replied, "Yes, I love those names. You can call me any of those." Little by little, the poopy talk dwindled away. By turning the *have to* of constant correction of name-calling into a *get to* of opportunities for creative brainstorming, I had goodified the poopy talk. I was pretty pleased with myself!

The Takeaway

This book contains dozens of stories from the field, scores of quotes from studies and experts, and hundreds of tips for overcoming burnout as an early childhood education professional. It's a lot to take in, and it's impossible to remember everything. So I'd like to leave you with three simple instructions. If you recall nothing else, I hope you'll remember these: Be joyful. Be present. And remember that your work is important.

Be joyful. Young children need joyful connections and trusting relationships with loving adults. They deserve this. They will not get it if there is negativity in the workplace and low morale.

Be present. When you are with a person, be with them fully. Being with a person fully means that the person has your full attention. You put your phone down. You might even silence it. You do not allow yourself to be distracted by a text or a social media notification. Nor do you try to multitask. Michael Formica urges us to recognize that "try as we might, we really can only do one thing at a time, so we ought to do that thing wholeheartedly. Most of our time is spent in the past or the future, rather than the present moment. What we end up doing is passing through that moment on the way to somewhere else and, in doing so, we miss the moment. That's how life ends up passing us by—we do it to ourselves" (Formica 2011). If you are a director and a teacher comes to you with a concern, stop and pay full attention, with eye contact and without the distraction of phones or computers. When a parent approaches for a conversation or a conference, try to do the same. If it is not an appropriate time for the discussion, find a time that allows full attention to their concerns.

Remember that your work is important. As a caregiver and teacher of young children, you are doing *the* most important job. You are nurturing, loving, creating mindful spaces, and building the brains of future mechanics, doctors, architects, social workers, firefighters, and politicians. You must fight against burnout by caring for yourself and finding balance in your career and your life.

• •

Reflection

- What are some household tasks you dislike doing? Write them down as *have tos*. (I have to _____.) Name as many as you want.

- Change the wording of these tasks. (I get to _____.)

- What are some ways to goodify these tasks? Think about timing yourself or inventing a cooperative game or competition with your spouse or child.

- What is a change you want to make? Think about paperwork, meetings, documentation, behaviors, lateness, and so on.

- Who are the people affected?

- Where does the change need to take place? Is it a change in policy, classroom, staff meetings?

- Name the good aspects of the needed change. (For example, why is that pesky documentation a good thing?)

- What are the not-so-great aspects? (For example, documentation takes so much time, and you have no planning time.)

- What is the overall goal that you want to achieve?

- How can you goodify this task to help you succeed? (For example, when I have a lot of computer documentation to do, I do it at a coffee shop so I can enjoy a latte while I work.)

Appendixes

Appendix A:
Program Wish List

Dear Families:

We aim to be frugal and use recycled, reused, and refurbished materials. If you come across any of the following items while you are recycling or grocery shopping or going to garage sales, our classroom will gratefully accept your donation.

1. _____

2. _____

3. _____

4. _____

5. _____

6. _____

7. _____

8. _____

9. _____

10. _____

11. _____

12. _____

13. _____

14. _____

15. _____

16. _____

17. _____

18. _____

19. _____

20. _____

21. _____

22. _____

23. _____

24. _____

25. _____

26. _____

27. _____

28. _____

29. _____

30. _____

Appendix B:
Individual Professional Development Plan

What are your current skills?

_____

_____

_____

_____

_____

_____

_____

What do you want to know more about?

_____

_____

_____

_____

_____

_____

_____

What are your professional goals for the next year?

_____

_____

_____

_____

_____

_____

What are your professional goals for the next five years?

_____

_____

_____

_____

_____

_____

Appendix C:
Physical Program and Classroom Improvements

How is your classroom meeting the goals of individual children?

_____

_____

_____

_____

_____

_____

Is the current environment working for the teachers _and_ the children? If not, why?

_____

_____

_____

_____

_____

_____

How can you make your classroom more accessible and more streamlined?

_____

_____

_____

_____

_____

_____

What tools do you use to make decisions about your classroom? For example, do you use the _Early Childhood Environmental Rating Scale_ (ECERS), the _Family Child Care Environmental Rating Scale_ (FCCERS), NAEYC accreditation standards, NAFCC quality standards, or other tools?

_____

_____

_____

_____

How often do you make physical changes in the classroom?

_____

_____

Do adjustments make your work harder or easier? Why?

_____

_____

_____

_____

_____

Is there time in your schedule to decide when change is needed? If not, how could you make time?

_____

_____

_____

_____

_____

_____

_____

When was the last time you changed your classroom?

_____

_____

What makes a classroom pleasing to you as a teacher?

_____

_____

_____

_____

_____

_____

What makes a classroom pleasing to a child?

_____

_____

_____

_____

_____

What makes a space overwhelming to teachers and children?

_____

_____

_____

_____

_____

_____

_____

Create a plan for each area of your classroom to get the environment you want. Make sure to take before and after photos.

_____

_____

_____

_____

_____

_____

_____

_____

Are there any items you need before you can start or finish this task? What are they?

_____

_____

_____

_____

_____

_____

What are your priorities?

_____

_____

_____

_____

_____

What needs to happen first?

_____

_____

_____

Appendix D:
Discussion Questions

The following questions are meant to guide conversation between child care providers that may be feeling the burnout described throughout *Overcoming Teacher Burnout*. To get the best experience from these questions, we encourage you to follow a few guidelines.

Facilitators are a great tool to use in discussions. The facilitator's role is not that of an expert or a participant, but as a guiding force of conversation. The facilitator should observe the dynamics in the group and respond to make sure all members of the group feel included in the discussion. The facilitator should make their role in the conversation known to the participants.

Conversations around this subject matter can take a lot of time out of the day if participants let it. It is important to establish the amount of time that the group wants to participate. The facilitator should also watch the clock and move conversation so each question holds roughly the same amount of time.

In this space, all members should feel that their experiences and opinions are valid. Promote a healthy environment by informing the group of this rule before discussion begins. Also, encourage listening and responses between the group members. Organic conversation is a wonderful way to dive deeper into these topics and spark a productive discussion.

1. Which story was the hardest to read or affected you the most? Why?

2. How is burnout different for child care providers than people in other professions?

3. How has burnout affected you as a provider?

4. Can burnout be solved or only managed?

5. What mistakes do you think you have made in your profession? Why do you hold on to them?

6. How do you typically react to complicated, stressful situations? Why do you react this way?

7. Are you a people person or a people pleaser?

8. How do you seek out feedback?

9. Where in your day-to-day job do you feel joy?

10. What was your favorite quote?

11. How can you take ownership of your continuous learning?

12. Are there ways to help a provider in the early stages of burnout while still practicing self-care?

13. Who in your life builds you up?

14. What is the most important thing in your life?

15. How can you goodify your day?

16. What happens when you leave your comfort zone?

17. What do you need to move forward in your career?

References

Ali, Titilayo Tinubu. 2016. "Strengthening the Early Childhood Workforce to Assure High-Quality Early Education." *Learning Policy Institute* (blog). August 12. https://learningpolicyinstitute.org/blog/strengthening-early-childhood-workforce-assure-high-quality-early-education.

Carter, Sherrie Bourg. 2012. "Why Mess Causes Stress: 8 Reasons, 8 Remedies." *Psychology Today*. March 14. www.psychologytoday.com/us/blog/high-octane-women/201203/why-mess-causes-stress-8-reasons-8-remedies.

CEI (Center for Educational Innovation). 2018. "Writing a Teaching Philosophy." University of Minnesota. Accessed October 8. https://cei.umn.edu/writing-your-teaching-philosophy.

Center on the Developing Child at Harvard University. 2007. *A Science-Based Framework for Early Childhood Policy: Using Evidence to Improve Outcomes in Learning, Behavior, and Health for Vulnerable Children*. https://developingchild.harvard.edu/resources/a-science-based-framework-for-early-childhood-policy.

CSCCE (Center for the Study of Child Care Employment). 2018. "Opportunity, Access, and Respect for Early Educators." http://cscce.berkeley.edu/opportunity-access-and-respect-for-early-educators/.

Concordia University–Portland. 2018. "Essential Trauma-Informed Teaching Strategies for Managing Stress in the Classroom." *Room 241* (blog). January 11. https://education.cu-portland.edu/blog/classroom-resources/trauma-informed-teaching-tips/.

Dickinson, Alexandra. 2017. "How to Say No without Feeling Guilty." *Forbes*. November 20. www.forbes.com/sites/alexandradickinson/2017/11/20/how-to-say-no-without-feeling-guilty/#386a93661bab.

Drolette, Ellen. 2016. "Sustaining High Staff Morale." *Exchange* 230 (July/August): 50–53.

Earthman, Glen I. and Linda K. Lemasters. 2009. "Teacher Attitudes about Classroom Conditions." *Journal of Educational Administration* 47 (3): 323–25.

Figley, Charles R. 1995. "Compassion Fatigue: Toward a New Understanding of the Costs of Caring." In *Secondary Traumatic Stress: Self-care Issues for Clinicians, Researchers, and Educators*, edited by B.H. Stamm, 3–28. Baltimore: The Sidran Press.

Fogg, B. J. 2013. "Fogg Method: 3 Steps to Changing Behavior." www.foggmethod.com.

Formica, Michael J. 2008. "Reframing Self Esteem as Self Worth." *Psychology Today* website. May 19. www.psychologytoday.com/us/blog/enlightened-living/200805/reframing-self-esteem-self-worth.

———. 2011. "5 Steps for Being Present." *Psychology Today*. June 14. www.psychologytoday.com/us/blog/enlightened-living/201106/5-steps-being-present.

Griffin, R. Morgan. 2008. "Give Your Body a Boost—with Laughter." WebMD. April 10. www.webmd.com/balance/features/give-your-body-boost-with-laughter#1.

Guarino, Cassandra, Lucrecia Santibañez, Glenn Daley, and Dominic Brewer. 2004. *A Review of the Research Literature on Teacher Recruitment and Retention*. Santa Monica, CA: Rand Corporation. www.rand.org/content/dam/rand/pubs/technical_reports/2005/RAND_TR164.pdf.

Heathfield, Susan M. 2018. "How to Deal with a Negative Coworker: Negativity Matters." *The Balance Careers* (blog). June 9. www.thebalancecareers.com/how-to-deal-with-a-negative-coworker-negativity-matters-1917875.

Hunter, Elaine. 2017. "How a Child's Brain Develops from the Womb to Age Five." *Theirworld* (blog). February 22. https://theirworld.org/news/how-childs-brain-develops-from-womb-to-age-five.

Institute of Medicine and the National Research Council. 2012. *The Early Childhood Care and Education Workforce: Challenges and Opportunities: A Workshop Report*. Washington, DC: National Academies Press. www.ncbi.nlm.nih.gov/books/NBK189908.

Jamison, Kay Redfield. 2004. *Exuberance: The Passion for Life*. New York: Vintage Books.

Life Is Good Company. 2018. "What We Do." https://content.lifeisgood.com/kidsfoundation/what-we-do.

Mead, Sara. 2018. "The Great Degree Debate." *U.S. News & World Report*. January 12. www.usnews.com/opinion/knowledge-bank/articles/2018-01-12/make-higher -education-more-accessible-to-early-childhood-teachers.

Miller, Donald. 2017. "The Brutal Cost of Overload and How to Reclaim the Rest You Need: Interview with Juliet Funt." *Building a Storybrand* podcast. April 17. http:// buildingastorybrand.com/episode-40.

NIMH (National Institute of Mental Health). 2017. "Mental Illness." Updated November 2017. www.nimh.nih.gov/health/statistics/mental-illness.shtml.

Patterson, James. 2001. *Suzanne's Diary for Nicholas*. New York: Warner Books.

Perry, Bruce D., and Maia Szalavitz. 2006. *The Boy Who Was Raised as a Dog and Other Stories from a Child Psychiatrist's Notebook: What Traumatized Children Can Teach Us about Loss, Love, and Healing*. New York: Basic Books.

Salmansohn, Karen. 2001. *How to Be Happy, Dammit: The Cynic's Guide to Spiritual Happiness*. New York: Celestial Arts.

Shaw, George Bernard. 1911. *The Doctor's Dilemma*. New York: Brentano's.

Smith, Anne B. 2014. "School Completion/Academic Achievement-Outcomes of Early Childhood Education." Encyclopedia on Early Childhood Development (website). May. www.child-encyclopedia.com/school-success/according-experts/school -completionacademic-achievement-outcomes-early-childhood.

Sussex Publishers. 2018. "Burnout." *Psychology Today*. Accessed April 24. www .psychologytoday.com/us/basics/burnout.

University of Missouri–Columbia. 2017. "Lack of Training Contributes to Burnout, Survey of Preschool Teachers Finds." *Phys.org* (blog). February 23. https://phys.org /news/2017-02-lack-contributes-burnout-survey-preschool.html.

Washington, Valora, Brenda Gadson, and Kathryn L. Amel. 2015. *The New Early Childhood Professional: A Step-by-Step Guide to Overcoming Goliath*. Washington, DC: Teachers College Press.

Whitaker, Robert C., Brandon D. Becker, Allison N. Herman, and Rachel A. Gooze. 2013. "The Physical and Mental Health of Head Start Staff: The Pennsylvania Head Start Staff Wellness Survey, 2012." *Preventing Chronic Disease* 10: E181. www.ncbi.nlm .nih.gov/pmc/articles/PMC3816599/.

Whitebook, Marcy, and Dan Bellm. 2014. "Mentors as Teachers, Learners, and Leaders." *Exchange* 218 (July/August): 14–18. http://cscce.berkeley.edu/files/2014 /FINAL-218-Whitebook-Bellm1.pdf.